Clinical Calculations for Nurses

With Basic Mathematics Review
Second Edition

PURDUE UNIVERSITY CALUMET,
DEPARTMENT OF NURSING
HAMMOND, IN 46323-2094

Clinical Calculations for Nurses

With Basic Mathematics Review
Second Edition

Mary Jane Cordón
Associate Professor of Mathematics
Pasadena City College
Pasadena, California

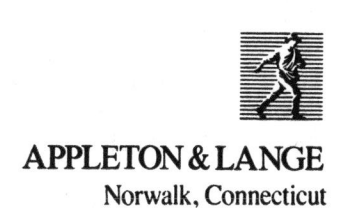

APPLETON & LANGE
Norwalk, Connecticut

0-8385-1214-3

Notice: Our knowledge in clinical sciences is constantly changing. As new information becomes available, changes in treatment and in the use of drugs become necessary. The author and the publisher of this volume have taken care to make certain that the doses of drugs and schedules of treatment are correct and compatible with the standards generally accepted at the time of publication. The reader is advised to consult carefully the instruction and information material included in the package insert of each drug or therapeutic agent before administration. This advice is especially important when using new or infrequently used drugs.

Copyright © 1990 by Appleton & Lange
A Publishing Division of Prentice Hall
Copyright © 1984 by Prentice-Hall, Inc., Englewood Cliffs, New Jersey

All rights reserved. This book, or any parts thereof, may not be used or reproduced in any manner without written permission. For information, address Appleton & Lange, 25 Van Zant Street, East Norwalk, Connecticut 06855.

90 91 92 93 94 / 10 9 8 7 6 5 4 3 2 1

Prentice Hall International (UK) Limited, *London*
Prentice Hall of Australia Pty. Limited, *Sydney*
Prentice Hall Canada, Inc., *Toronto*
Prentice Hall Hispanoamericana, S.A., *Mexico*
Prentice Hall of India Private Limited, *New Delhi*
Prentice Hall of Japan, Inc., *Tokyo*
Simon & Schuster Asia Pte. Ltd., *Singapore*
Editora Prentice Hall do Brasil Ltda., *Rio de Janeiro*
Prentice Hall, *Englewood Cliffs, New Jersey*

Library of Congress Cataloging-in-Publication Data

Cordón, Mary Jane.
  Clinical calculations for nurses : with basic mathematics review / Mary Jane Cordón.—2nd ed.
      p. cm.
  ISBN 0-8385-1214-3
  1. Pharmaceutical arithmetic.   2. Pharmaceutical arithmetic-
-Examinations, questions, etc.   3. Nursing—Mathematics.   I. Title.
  [DNLM: 1. Mathematics—nurses' instruction.   2. Mathematics-
-problems.   3. Pharmacology, Clinical—nurses' instruction.
4. Pharmacology, Clinical—problems.   QV 18 C796c]
RS57.C67 1989
615'.14—dc20
DNLM/DLC
for Library of Congress   89-6917
                                                             CIP

Acquisition Editor: Marion K. Welch
Production Editor: Susan Meiman
Cover Design: Michael Kelly

PRINTED IN THE UNITED STATES OF AMERICA

Contents

Preface / ix

Part I Basic Mathematics Review / 1

Diagnostic Test Basic Mathematics Review / 1

Chapter 1   Fractions and Mixed Numbers / 5

    Chapter 1 Pretest / *5*
    Objectives / *6*
    1.1 Definition of a Fraction / *7*
    1.2 Fractions and Mixed Numbers / *9*
    1.3 Operations with Fractions and Mixed Numbers / *13*
    1.4 Chapter Review Problems / *25*
    1.5 Chapter 1 Self Test / *27*

Chapter 2   Decimal Numbers / 32

    Chapter 2 Pretest / *32*
    Objectives / *33*
    2.1 Reading and Writing Decimal Numbers / *33*

2.2 Comparing and Rounding Off Decimal Numbers / *36*
2.3 Operations with Decimal Numbers / *40*
2.4 Converting Common Fractions and Mixed Numbers to Decimal Numbers; Changing Decimals to Fractions / *45*
2.5 Chapter 2 Review Problems / *47*
2.6 Chapter 2 Self Test / *49*

Chapter 3 Ratios, Proportions, and Percents / *53*

Chapter 3 Pretest / *53*
3.1 Ratios and Proportions / *54*
3.2 Solving Proportions / *58*
3.3 Converting a Percent to an Equivalent Decimal Form and a Decimal Form to an Equivalent Percent Form / *66*
3.4 The Percent Proportion / *68*
3.5 Chapter 3 Review Problems / *73*
3.6 Chapter 3 Self Test / *75*

Part II Clinical Calculations / 79

Chapter 4 The Metric System of Measurement / *79*

Objectives / *79*
Introduction / *79*
4.1 The Basic Metric Units of Measure / *80*
4.2 Metric Conversions / *84*
4.3 Temperature Scales / *89*
4.4 Metric Units and Their Applications / *92*
4.5 Chapter 4 Review Problems / *96*
4.6 Chapter 4 Self Test / *98*

Chapter 5 The Apothecaries' and Household Systems of Measurement and Conversions / *100*

Objectives / *100*
Introduction / *100*
5.1 Apothecaries' Units of Measure / *101*
5.2 The Household Units of Measure / *103*
5.3 Conversions From One Unit of Measure to Another / *104*

Contents   vii

    5.4 Applications Involving Apothecaries', Household, and Metric Units / *110*
    5.5 Chapter 5 Review Problems / *119*
    5.6 Chapter 5 Self Test / *122*

Chapter 6 Calculations for Oral and Parenteral Dosages / 125

    Objectives / *125*
    Introduction / *125*
    6.1 Calculating Dosages of Tablets and Capsules / *126*
    6.2 Calculating Dosages of Oral Solutions / *132*
    6.3 Calculating Dosages of Injectable Drugs / *138*
    6.4 Chapter 6 Review Problems / *147*
    6.5 Chapter 6 Self Test / *156*

Chapter 7 Calculations for Intravenous Fluids / 161

    Objectives / *161*
    Introduction / *161*
    7.1 Calculating the Rate of Flow / *162*
    7.2 Calculating the Running Time / *167*
    7.3 Piggyback IV's / *170*
    7.4 Chapter 7 Review Problems / *173*
    7.5 Chapter 7 Self Test / *175*

Chapter 8 Calculations for Pediatric Dosages / 177

    Objectives / *177*
    Introduction / *177*
    8.1 Calculating Pediatric Dosages Based on Body Surface / *177*
    8.2 Calculating Pediatric Dosages Based on Age and Body Mass / *182*
    8.3 Chapter 8 Review Problems / *185*
    8.4 Chapter 8 Self Test / *186*

Chapter 9 Computer-Generated Medication Administration Records / 189

    Objectives / *189*
    Introduction / *189*
    9.1 Twenty-Four-Hour Clock / *190*

9.2 Computer-Generated Medication Administration Records / *193*
9.3 Chapter 9 Review Problems / *200*
9.4 Chapter 9 Self Test / *201*

Chapter 10 Calculations for the Preparation of Solutions (Optional) / 204

Objectives / *204*
Introduction / *204*
10.1 Interpreting Solution Labels / *204*
10.2 Calculating the Amount of Pure Drug, Solvent, and Finished Solution / *208*
10.3 Calculating the Strength of a Solution / *216*
10.4 Preparing a Weak Solution From a Strong Solution / *220*
10.5 Chapter 10 Review Problems / *223*
10.6 Chapter 10 Self Test / *226*

Appendix I Roman Numerals / 230

Appendix II Commonly Used Medical Abbreviations / 234

Appendix III West Nomogram / 238

Appendix IV Final Exam Self Review / 240

Appendix V Answers / 247

Preface

The purpose of *Clinical Calculations for Nurses* is to aid nurses in applying basic mathematical concepts to on-the-job clinical situations.

The distinguishing aspects of this book are the easy-to-understand level of writing, the ratio-proportion approach to all the problems, the easily-detected, boxed rules, and the self-explanatory step-by-step examples. Students are carefully guided through each rule and example to minimize math anxiety. Newly introduced terms are highlighted in boldface type so they can be readily recognized. Problems are graduated in level of difficulty from simple to more complex. Actual drug orders written by a physician are used, and the actual drug labels are reproduced to give the students a sense of being in a real-life clinical situation.

The second edition of *Clinical Calculations for Nurses* contains a new chapter informing nursing students of the latest developments in computerized medication administration records. With the great efficiency and availability of computers, many hospitals have converted to a computerized system of generating medication administration records. Therefore, computer printouts of actual medical administration records have been incorporated into this chapter. Nursing students must not only be aware of these computer printouts, but must be able to interpret them if they intend to administer medications.

This text can be used in a traditional lecture class, in an individualized classroom situation, or in a learning center. (Videotape cassette lectures for some chapters are available from the author for use in a learning center.)

The book begins with Part I, a basic mathematics review of fractions, decimals, ratios, proportions, and percents. Chapters 1 through 3 enable students to review or restudy the basic mathematical concepts encountered by nurses and thus alleviate much math anxiety connected with the course. The Part I math section begins with a diagnostic math test in which students can ascertain their own math readiness. All the test questions are correlated with the first three chapters of the book so that students can identify, in general, their own areas of math deficiencies. Each of these chapters has a pretest so that the students can exactly pinpoint the chapter section they need to study. Students should review all weak areas before proceeding to Chapter 4.

Part II, Clinical Calculations, begins by introducing the students in Chapters 4 and 5 to the three systems of measure: the metric system, apothecaries' system, and the household system. The text integrates the basic math concepts and the systems of measure into clinical situations. Chapter 6 teaches how to calculate oral and parenteral dosages; Chapter 7 shows the calculations for intravenous fluids; and Chapter 8 demonstrates the calculations for pediatric dosages; Chapter 9 teaches how to read computerized medication administration records; and Chapter 10 shows how to prepare solutions.

Chapters 4 through 10 each have the following components:

1. Student objectives
2. Introduction of the topic
3. Explanation of the topic with precise rules
4. Detailed step-by-step examples
5. Practice problems after each chapter section
6. Chapter review problems
7. Referenced chapter self test

The chapter self test is referenced to chapter sections so that students can easily pinpoint areas of weakness and identify chapter sections to be restudied. The answers to all the practice problems and chapter reviews are in back of the text to enable the students to self check their work. The appendix includes a final exam self review for the benefit of the students.

In addition to the new chapter on computerized medication administration records, the following changes have also been incorporated in the text.

1. Chapter 6, from the first edition, is Chapter 9 in the second edition. Since this chapter on solutions is not taught in some nursing programs, it can now be an optional chapter for the course.
2. The formulas for calculating pediatric dosages have been rewritten. These new formulas make the calculations easier for the students.

The answers to the chapter self tests and the final exam review are printed in the Instructor's Manual. The instructor can use these self tests as a checkpoint to measure the students' progress, or the instructor can provide these answers to the students for self-checking. The Instructor's Manual also contains two forms of achievement tests for each chapter, two forms of a final exam, and the answers to all these tests.

Special thanks go to Huntington Memorial Hospital, Kaiser Permanente Hospital, and Glendale Adventist Hospital for sharing their information on computer generated medication administration records.

Also, thanks to Neville Williams, M.D., for writing prescriptions used in this text, Eli Lilly and Company; and Merck, Sharp, and Dohme, Division of Merck and Company, for permission to reproduce their drug labels. Lastly, thanks to Marion K. Welch, Acquisition Editor, and Susan Meiman, Production Editor, for their support and encouragement in printing this second edition.

Mary Jane Cordón

PART I Basic Mathematics Review

Diagnostic Test
Basic Mathematics Review

Chapter 1. Perform the operations. *Reduce* all answers to lowest terms. Change improper fractions to mixed numbers.

1. $39 - \dfrac{3}{10} =$ 1. _____

2. $2\dfrac{1}{2} - 1\dfrac{9}{16} =$ 2. _____

3. $5\dfrac{1}{3} + 6\dfrac{1}{18} + 3\dfrac{1}{4} =$ 3. _____

4. $3\dfrac{3}{4} \times 2\dfrac{1}{10} =$ 4. _____

5. $2\dfrac{3}{4} \div 2\dfrac{1}{16} =$ 5. _____

Chapter 2. Change each fraction to an equivalent decimal number. *Round off each answer to the nearest tenth.*

6. $\dfrac{5}{16}$ _____   7. $\dfrac{5}{4}$ _____

1

8. $\dfrac{5}{6}$ _____   9. $\dfrac{2}{9}$ _____

10. $\dfrac{12}{5}$ _____

Chapter 2. Perform the operations.

11. $28.37 - 19.189 =$ 11. _____

12. $11.35 - 1.19 + 0.638 - 2.5103 =$ 12. _____

13. $2.004 \times 1.08 =$ 13. _____

14. $4.005 - 0.75 =$ 14. _____

15. $585 \div 0.13 =$ 15. _____

Chapter 3. Change each decimal number to an equivalent percent.

16. 0.0033 _____   17. 0.9 _____

18. 0.04 _____   19. 6.5 _____

20. 0.425 _____

Chapter 3. Change each percent to an equivalent decimal number.

21. 0.0025% _____   22. 5.8% _____

23. $3\dfrac{1}{2}\%$ _____   24. 0.9% _____

25. 315% _____

Chapter 3. Solve for x in each of the following proportions.

26. $\dfrac{\frac{1}{8}}{1} = \dfrac{\frac{1}{24}}{x}$ 26. _____

27. $\dfrac{\frac{1}{250}}{x} = \dfrac{5}{100}$ 27. _____

Diagnostic Test, Basic Mathematics Review

28. $\dfrac{1.5}{1} = \dfrac{1350}{x}$ 28. _____

29. $\dfrac{x}{\frac{1}{3}} = \dfrac{120}{\frac{1}{2}}$ 29. _____

30. $\dfrac{1}{20{,}000} = \dfrac{x}{350}$ 30. _____

Chapter 3. Change each of the following ratios to its decimal equivalent.

31. 1:200 _____   32. $\dfrac{1}{150}$ _____

33. $\dfrac{1}{9}$ _____   34. 1:5000 _____

35. 1:8 _____

Chapter 3. Solve each of the following.

36. Find 150% of 3.56.   36. _____

37. Find $4\dfrac{1}{2}$% of 86 kg.   37. _____

38. 60 is 45% of what number?   38. _____

39. 15 is 80% of what number?   39. _____

40. 45 is what percent of 120?   40. _____

Chapter 3. Which one is greater?

41. 0.02% or 0.1%   41. _____

42. 0.0033% or 0.025%   42. _____

43. 1:200 or 5%   43. _____

44. 0.025% or 1:400   44. _____

45. 1:400 or 2:300   45. _____

Chapters 1 and 2. Simplify.

46. $\dfrac{1000 \times 20}{4 \times 60} =$ 46. _____

47. $\dfrac{1000 \times 15}{10 \times 60} =$ 47. _____

48. $\dfrac{5}{150} \times 9000 =$ 48. _____

49. $\dfrac{8.5}{20} \times 240 =$ 49. _____

50. $\dfrac{0.86}{1.72} \times 4 =$ 50. _____

1
Fractions and Mixed Numbers

PRETEST

Chapter
Section

1.1   **1.** Shade $\dfrac{5}{16}$ of the rectangle.

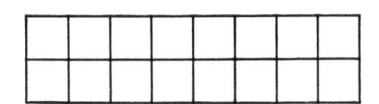

1.2   **2.** Change $\dfrac{48}{14}$ to a mixed number reduced to lowest terms. _____

1.2   **3.** Change $6\dfrac{9}{11}$ to an improper fraction. _____

1.2   **4.** Reduce $\dfrac{72}{84}$ to lowest terms. _____

1.2   **5.** Change $\dfrac{5}{13}$ to an equivalent fraction having 65 as its denominator. _____

1.3   6. State the reciprocal of $\dfrac{3}{11}$. _____

1.3   7. Find the least common denominator (LCD) for $\dfrac{1}{12}$, $\dfrac{1}{14}$, and $\dfrac{1}{15}$.
_____

Perform the following operations. Reduce all answers to lowest terms. Change all improper fractions to mixed numbers.

1.3   8. $\dfrac{3}{8} + \dfrac{5}{12} =$ _____

1.3   9. $\dfrac{5}{6} - \dfrac{3}{9} =$ _____

1.3   10. $3\dfrac{1}{10} + 1\dfrac{3}{15} =$ _____

1.3   11. $8\dfrac{5}{8} - 5\dfrac{11}{12} =$ _____

1.3   12. $4\dfrac{1}{2} \times 6\dfrac{2}{3} =$ _____

1.3   13. $\dfrac{6}{25} \div 3 =$ _____

1.3   14. $\dfrac{8}{13} \times \dfrac{39}{40} \times \dfrac{5}{9} =$ _____

1.3   15. $2\dfrac{4}{15} \div 2\dfrac{11}{20} =$ _____

OBJECTIVES

After studying this chapter you should be able to

1. read and write common fractions;
2. change improper fractions to mixed numbers and mixed numbers to improper fractions;
3. change a given fraction to an equivalent fraction;

1.1. Definition of a Fraction

4. reduce fractions to lowest terms;
5. find the least common denominator for fractions with unlike denominators;
6. add, subtract, multiply, and divide fractions and mixed numbers.

1.1 DEFINITION OF A FRACTION

A whole unit may be divided into equal parts. The equal parts of a whole are represented by a **common fraction**.

The circle shown has been divided into two equal fractional parts.

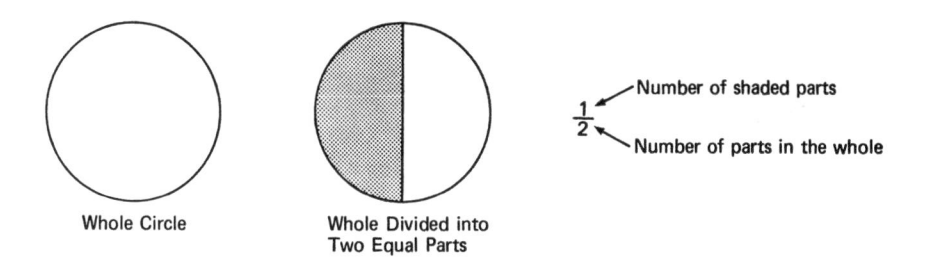

$\frac{1}{2}$ ← Number of shaded parts
← Number of parts in the whole

Whole Circle

Whole Divided into Two Equal Parts

The rectangle shown has been divided into three equal fractional parts.

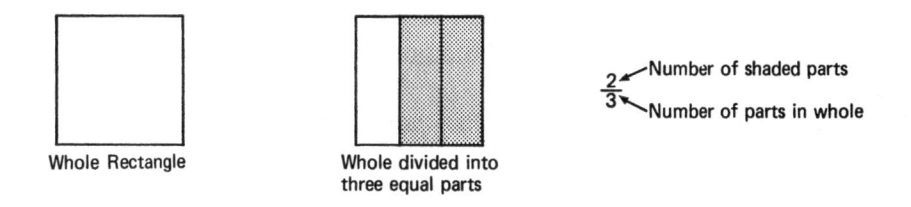

$\frac{2}{3}$ ← Number of shaded parts
← Number of parts in whole

Whole Rectangle

Whole divided into three equal parts

A **common fraction** is written in the form $\frac{a}{b}$. a and b ($b \neq 0$) are called the **terms** of the fraction. b, the number below the fraction bar, called the **denominator**, designates into how many parts the whole has been divided. a, the number above the fraction bar, called the **numerator**, designates the number of parts talked about or used.

Fraction bar → $\frac{a}{b}$ → Numerator
← Denominator (cannot be zero)

PRACTICE SET 1.1

1. Write the fraction for the shaded parts of the figures.

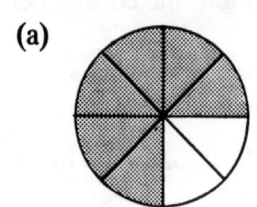

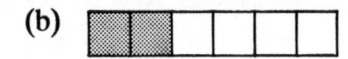

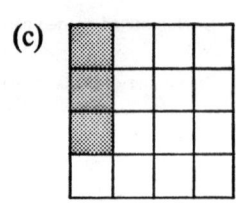

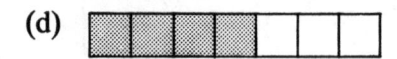

    (a)

    (b)

    (c)

    (d)

2. If five equal parts of a figure are shaded, and there are twelve equal parts altogether, what number should be used as the numerator of the fraction representing the number *not* shaded?

3. In the fraction $\frac{4}{9}$, name the numerator and the denominator.

4. Shade the parts of each figure corresponding to the fraction.

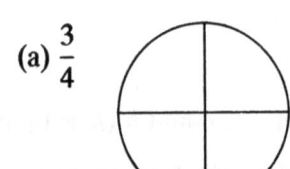

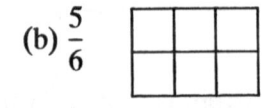

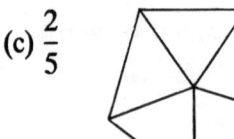

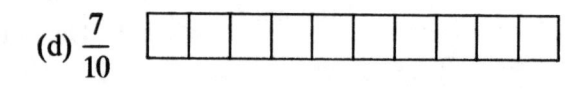

    (a) $\frac{3}{4}$

    (b) $\frac{5}{6}$

    (c) $\frac{2}{5}$

    (d) $\frac{7}{10}$

5. Write a fraction for the part of the glass that has water in it.

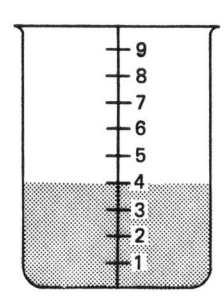

1.2 FRACTIONS AND MIXED NUMBERS

A **proper fraction** is a fraction whose numerator is smaller than its denominator. Some examples are:

$$\frac{1}{2}, \frac{3}{4}, \frac{5}{6}, \frac{7}{9}, \frac{6}{11}$$

An **improper fraction** is a fraction whose numerator is greater than or equal to its denominator. Some examples are:

$$\frac{5}{4}, \frac{4}{3}, \frac{9}{5}, \frac{11}{5}, \frac{8}{8}$$

A **mixed number** is a number having a whole number part and a fraction part. Some examples of mixed numbers are:

$$1\frac{1}{4}, 6\frac{3}{5}, 7\frac{1}{2}, 3\frac{3}{8}$$

Improper fractions can be changed to mixed numbers.

RULE 1.1 Rule to Change an Improper Fraction to a Mixed Number

Step 1. Divide the numerator by the denominator.

Step 2. Write this quotient followed by the fraction: $\frac{\text{remainder}}{\text{divisor}}$.

EXAMPLE 1.1

Change the following improper fractions to mixed numbers.

(a) $\frac{16}{3}$ **Step 1.**   **Step 2.**

$$3\overline{\smash{)}16} \atop \underline{15} \atop 1 }^{5} = 5\frac{1}{3} \begin{array}{l} \leftarrow \text{Remainder} \\ \leftarrow \text{Divisor} \end{array}$$

Quotient

Answer. $\frac{16}{3} = 5\frac{1}{3}$

(b) $\frac{21}{6}$ **Step 1.**   **Step 2.**

$$6\overline{\smash{)}21} \atop \underline{18} \atop 3 }^{3} = 3\frac{3}{6} \begin{array}{l} \leftarrow \text{Remainder} \\ \leftarrow \text{Divisor} \end{array}$$

Quotient

Answer. $\frac{21}{6} = 3\frac{3}{6}$

A mixed number can be converted to an improper fraction.

RULE 1.2   Rule for Changing a Mixed Number to an Improper Fraction

Step 1. Multiply the denominator by the whole number.

Step 2. Add the numerator to the product obtained in Step 1.

Step 3. Write the sum from Step 2 as the numerator in a fraction. The denominator is the denominator of the original fraction.

EXAMPLE 1.2

Change the following mixed numbers to improper fractions.

(a) $2\frac{3}{4}$

   Step 1. $4 \times 2 = 8$

   Step 2. $8 + 3 = 11$

1.2. Fractions and Mixed Numbers

Step 3. $\dfrac{11}{4}$ ← Sum
← Original denominator

Answer. $2\dfrac{3}{4} = \dfrac{11}{4}$

(b) $3\dfrac{1}{5}$

Step 1. $5 \times 3 = 15$

Step 2. $15 + 1 = 16$

Step 3. $\dfrac{16}{5}$ ← Sum
← Original denominator

Answer. $3\dfrac{1}{5} = \dfrac{16}{5}$

The same number can be represented by many different fractional numerals. Two fractional numerals representing the same number are called **equivalent fractions**. An equivalent fraction can be formed by multiplying the given fraction by any fractional form of 1, excluding $\dfrac{1}{1}$.

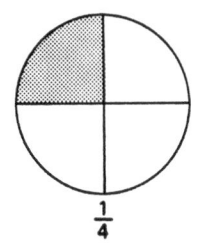

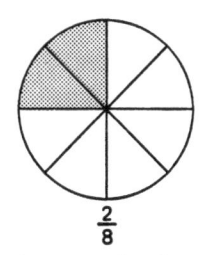

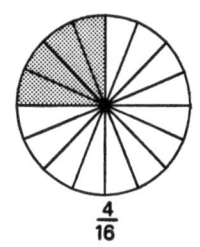

$$\dfrac{1}{4} = \dfrac{2}{8} = \dfrac{4}{16}$$

Equivalent Fractions

EXAMPLE 1.3

(a) $\dfrac{1}{2} \times \dfrac{4}{4} = \dfrac{4}{8}$ ← Equivalent fraction for $\dfrac{1}{2}$
↑
Fractional form of 1

Answer. $\dfrac{1}{2} = \dfrac{4}{8}$

(b) $\dfrac{3}{4} \times \dfrac{2}{2} = \dfrac{6}{8}$ ← Equivalent fraction for $\dfrac{3}{4}$

↑
Fractional form of 1

Answer. $\dfrac{3}{4} = \dfrac{6}{8}$

A fraction can also be changed to an equivalent fraction by dividing both the numerator and the denominator by the same common factor. The **greatest common factor** of two numbers is the largest number that evenly divides the two given numbers. The process of changing a fraction to an equivalent fraction by dividing the numerator and the denominator by the greatest common factor is called **reducing a fraction to lowest terms.**

RULE 1.3 Rule for Reducing Fractions to Lowest Terms

Divide both the numerator and the denominator by the greatest common factor.

EXAMPLE 1.4

Reduce each of the following fractions to lowest terms.

(a) $\dfrac{14}{21}$

$\dfrac{14 \div 7}{21 \div 7} = \dfrac{2}{3}$ ← Reduced fraction

↑
Divide the numerator and denominator by the greatest common factor, 7.

Answer. $\dfrac{14}{21} = \dfrac{2}{3}$

(b) $\dfrac{15}{40}$

$\dfrac{15 \div 5}{40 \div 5} = \dfrac{3}{8}$ ← Reduced fraction

Answer. $\dfrac{15}{40} = \dfrac{3}{8}$

1.3. Operations with Fractions and Mixed Numbers

PRACTICE SET 1.2

1. Find the improper fractions among the following.
$$\frac{16}{3}, \frac{1}{4}, \frac{8}{9}, \frac{5}{5}, \frac{11}{4}$$

2. Change the following improper fractions to mixed numbers.
$$\frac{9}{2}, \frac{16}{3}, \frac{32}{11}, \frac{8}{7}, \frac{16}{5}$$

3. Change the following mixed numbers to improper fractions.
$$2\frac{1}{4}, 1\frac{7}{8}, 5\frac{1}{2}, 6\frac{1}{4}, 8\frac{3}{4}$$

4. Change each given fraction to an equivalent fraction as indicated.
   (a) $\frac{1}{2} \times \frac{5}{5} =$ (b) $\frac{3}{8} \times \frac{9}{9} =$ (c) $\frac{4}{5} \times \frac{25}{25} =$

5. Reduce each of the following fractions to lowest terms.
   (a) $\frac{6}{9}$ (b) $\frac{21}{56}$ (c) $\frac{66}{99}$

1.3 OPERATIONS WITH FRACTIONS AND MIXED NUMBERS

Two fractions having the same denominator are said to have a **common denominator.** Fractions with the same denominator can be added or subtracted.

RULE 1.4 Rule for Adding or Subtracting Fractions with Common Denominators

Step 1. Add or subtract the numerators.

Step 2. Write the sum or the difference as the numerator of a fraction and the common denominator as the denominator.

Step 3. Reduce the fraction to lowest terms. Change all improper fractions to mixed numbers.

EXAMPLE 1.5

(a) $\quad \dfrac{5}{8} + \dfrac{7}{8} = \quad \dfrac{12}{8} \quad = 1\dfrac{4}{8} = \quad 1\dfrac{1}{2}$

↑ Add numerators   ↑ Sum written with same denominator   ↑ Reduced fraction

(b) $\dfrac{9}{16} - \dfrac{1}{16} = \dfrac{8}{16} = \dfrac{1}{2}$
   ↑   ↑   ↑
Subtract   Difference   Reduced
numerators with same   fraction
            denominator

Mixed numbers are treated in the same manner as fractions. Add or subtract the fraction part separately from the whole number part. Then add or subtract the whole numbers.

EXAMPLE 1.6

(a) $\begin{array}{r} 1\dfrac{3}{4} \\ +\ 2\dfrac{2}{4} \\ \hline \end{array}\ \Rightarrow\ \begin{array}{r} 1\dfrac{3}{4} \\ +\ 2\dfrac{2}{4} \\ \hline 3\dfrac{5}{4} \end{array}$ ← Change improper fraction to mixed number.

$$3 \quad \dfrac{5}{4}$$
$$\downarrow \quad \downarrow$$
$$3 + 1\dfrac{1}{4} = 4\dfrac{1}{4}$$
$$\uparrow$$
$$\text{Add}$$

Answer. $1\dfrac{3}{4} + 2\dfrac{2}{4} = 4\dfrac{1}{4}$

(b) $\begin{array}{r} 7\dfrac{5}{9} \\ -\ 2\dfrac{2}{9} \\ \hline \end{array}\ \Rightarrow\ \begin{array}{r} 7\dfrac{5}{9} \\ -\ 2\dfrac{2}{9} \\ \hline 5\dfrac{3}{9} = 5\dfrac{1}{3} \end{array}$ ← Reduced fraction

Answer. $7\dfrac{5}{9} - 2\dfrac{2}{9} = 5\dfrac{1}{3}$

1.3. Operations with Fractions and Mixed Numbers

Sometimes it is not possible to subtract mixed numbers as they are written. The mixed numbers may be changed to improper fractions so that subtraction can be performed.

EXAMPLE 1.7

(a) $\quad 5\frac{1}{4} \quad \Rightarrow \quad \frac{21}{4} \quad \leftarrow$ Mixed numbers changed

$\quad\quad -2\frac{3}{4} \quad\quad\quad -\frac{11}{4} \quad \swarrow$ to improper fractions

$$\frac{10}{4} = 2\frac{2}{4} = 2\frac{1}{2} \leftarrow \text{Reduced fraction}$$

Answer. $\quad 5\frac{1}{4} - 2\frac{3}{4} = 2\frac{1}{2}$

(b) $\quad 6\frac{2}{8} \quad \Rightarrow \quad \frac{50}{8}$

$\quad\quad -1\frac{5}{8} \quad\quad\quad -\frac{13}{8}$

$$\frac{37}{8} = 4\frac{5}{8}$$

Answer. $\quad 6\frac{2}{8} - 1\frac{5}{8} = 4\frac{5}{8}$

Fractions with different denominators must be converted to equivalent fractions having the same denominator before they can be added or subtracted. This requires finding the **least common denominator** (LCD).

For example:

$$\frac{5}{12} + \frac{7}{24}$$

cannot be added until the least common denominator is found and both fractions converted to equivalent fractions with the least common denominator as their denominators. The least common denominator in the example cited is 24 because both 12 and 24 divide into 24 evenly. Finding the LCD involves finding prime numbers that are common factors of the denominators. A **prime number** is a number greater than one that has only the factors 1 and itself.

5 is a prime number because the numbers 1 and 5 are its only factors.

13 is a prime number because the numbers 1 and 13 are its only factors.

A **prime factor** is a prime number that divides exactly into another number. For example:

5 is a prime factor of 15 because it is a prime number that divides exactly into 15; 3 is the other prime factor of 15.

7 is a prime factor of 21 because it is a prime number that divides exactly into 21; 3 is the other prime factor of 21.

11 is a prime factor of 44 because it is a prime number that divides exactly into 44; 2 is the other prime factor of 44. Note that 4 is not a prime factor of 44 because 4 is not a prime number.

RULE 1.5 Rule for Finding the Least Common Denominator (LCD)

Step 1. Write the denominators in a horizontal line.

Step 2. Find a prime factor that divides exactly into at least two of the denominators. Write the quotients on the line below.

Step 3. Any denominator not divided exactly by the prime factor is brought down to the line below.

Step 4. Repeat this division step until no prime number divides at least two denominators on the quotient line.

Step 5. Multiply all the prime factors by all the numbers on the last quotient line.

EXAMPLE 1.8

Find the LCD for $\dfrac{1}{6}, \dfrac{5}{12}, \dfrac{7}{24}$.

Step 1.   6   12   24   ← Write the denominators in a horizontal line.

Steps 2–3. 2 | 6   12   24   ← 2 is a prime factor that divides into the three
              3   6   12   numbers evenly. Write the quotients on the line below.

Step 4.   2 | 6   12   24   ← Continue the process of Step 2 dividing each
              3 | 3   6   12   quotient line by 3 and 2.
              2 | 1   2   4   ← Since 2 does not divide into 1 evenly, write the 1 on
                  1   1   2   the quotient line.

Step 5. LCD = 2 × 3 × 2 × 1 × 1 × 2 = 24

Answer. The LCD = 24

1.3. Operations with Fractions and Mixed Numbers

EXAMPLE 1.9

Find the LCD for $\frac{1}{14}$, $\frac{1}{15}$, and $\frac{1}{18}$.

Step 1. 14 15 18

Steps 2–4.
$$\begin{array}{r|rrr} 2 & 14 & 15 & 18 \\ 3 & 7 & 15 & 9 \\ \hline & 7 & 5 & 3 \end{array}$$

Step 5. LCD = 2 × 3 × 7 × 5 × 3 = 630

Answer. The LCD = 630

RULE 1.6 Rule for Adding and Subtracting Fractions with Unlike Denominators

Step 1. Find the LCD.

Step 2. Convert each fraction to an equivalent fraction having the LCD as its denominator.

Step 3. Add or subtract the fractions.

Step 4. Reduce the answer to lowest terms. Change improper fractions to mixed numbers.

EXAMPLE 1.10

$\frac{1}{4} + \frac{1}{18} =$

Step 1. Find the LCD.

$$\begin{array}{r|rr} 2 & 4 & 18 \\ & 2 & 9 \end{array}$$

LCD = 2 × 2 × 9

LCD = 36

Step 2. Convert each fraction to an equivalent fraction with the LCD as its denominator.

$$\frac{1}{4} = \frac{9}{36}$$

$$\frac{1}{18} = \frac{2}{36}$$

Step 3. Add the fractions.
$$\frac{9}{36} + \frac{2}{36} = \frac{11}{36}$$

Step 4. $\frac{11}{36}$ is in lowest terms.

Answer. $\frac{1}{4} + \frac{1}{18} = \frac{11}{36}$

EXAMPLE 1.11

$$\frac{6}{12} - \frac{3}{14} =$$

Step 1. Find the LCD.

LCD = 2 × 6 × 7 = 84

$$\begin{array}{r|rr} 2 & 12 & 14 \\ & 6 & 7 \end{array}$$

Step 2. Convert each fraction to an equivalent fraction.
$$\frac{6}{12} = \frac{42}{84}$$
$$\frac{3}{14} = \frac{18}{84}$$

Step 3. Subtract.
$$\frac{42}{84} - \frac{18}{84} = \frac{24}{84}$$

Step 4. Reduce to lowest terms.
$$\frac{24}{84} \div \frac{12}{12} = \frac{2}{7}$$

Answer. $\frac{6}{12} - \frac{3}{14} = \frac{2}{7}$

Mixed numbers containing unlike fractions can be added or subtracted using the same rule.

EXAMPLE 1.12

$$5\frac{1}{4} + 3\frac{1}{5} + 2\frac{1}{12} =$$

1.3. Operations with Fractions and Mixed Numbers

Step 1. Find the LCD.

LCD = 2 × 2 × 1 × 5 × 3

LCD = 60

```
2 | 4  5  12
2 | 2  5   6
    1  5   3
```

Step 2. Convert each fraction to an equivalent fraction.

$$5\frac{1}{4} = 5\frac{15}{60}$$
$$3\frac{1}{5} = 3\frac{12}{60}$$
$$2\frac{1}{12} = 2\frac{5}{60}$$

Step 3. Add. $10\frac{32}{60}$

Step 4. Reduce. $10\frac{32}{60} = 10\frac{8}{15}$

Answer. $5\frac{1}{4} + 3\frac{1}{5} + 2\frac{1}{12} = 10\frac{8}{15}$

To multiply fractions, multiply the numerators, multiply the denominators, and reduce the resulting fraction to lowest terms. Improper fractions may be converted to mixed numbers.

RULE 1.7 Rule for Multiplying Fractions

Step 1. Multiply numerators.

Step 2. Multiply denominators.

Step 3. Write the product of the numerators as the numerator of your answer and write the product of the denominators as the denominator of your answer.

Step 4. Reduce the fraction. Change the improper fractions to mixed numbers.

EXAMPLE 1.13

(a) $\dfrac{3}{5} \times \dfrac{2}{7} = \dfrac{6}{35}$

(b) $\dfrac{1}{2} \times \dfrac{5}{8} \times \dfrac{2}{5} = \dfrac{10}{80} = \dfrac{1}{8}$

The operation of multiplication can be simplified by means of a process called **cancelling**; that is, fractions in a multiplication problem can be reduced prior to multiplication. Any one numerator and any one denominator can be divided by the same common factor.

EXAMPLE 1.14

$$\frac{7}{12} \times \frac{3}{30} =$$

Step 1. Divide 3 and 12 by 3.
Step 2. Divide 7 and 21 by 7.

Answer.
$$\frac{7}{12} \times \frac{3}{21} = \frac{1}{12}$$

EXAMPLE 1.15

$$\frac{24}{55} \times \frac{35}{36} \times \frac{11}{28} =$$

Step 1. Divide 11 and 55 by 11.
Step 2. Divide 24 and 36 by 12.
Step 3. Divide 35 and 5 by 5.
Step 4. Divide 7 and 28 by 7.
Step 5. Divide 2 and 4 by 2.

Answer.
$$\frac{24}{55} \times \frac{35}{36} \times \frac{11}{28} = \frac{1}{6}$$

RULE 1.8 Rule for Multiplying Mixed Numbers

Step 1. Change each mixed number to an equivalent improper fraction.

Step 2. Multiply the fractions. Cancel if possible.

Step 3. Reduce the fraction. Change any improper fraction to a mixed number.

EXAMPLE 1.16

$$2\frac{1}{2} \times 3\frac{3}{4} =$$

1.3. Operations with Fractions and Mixed Numbers   21

Step 1. $\dfrac{5}{2} \times \dfrac{15}{4} =$

Step 2. $\dfrac{5}{2} \times \dfrac{15}{4} = \dfrac{75}{8}$

Step 3. $\dfrac{75}{8} = 9\dfrac{3}{8}$

Answer. $2\dfrac{1}{2} \times 3\dfrac{3}{4} = 9\dfrac{3}{8}$

EXAMPLE 1.17

$5\dfrac{1}{2} \times 12 =$

Step 1. $\dfrac{11}{2} \times \dfrac{12}{1} =$

Steps 2 and 3. $\dfrac{11}{\cancel{2}_1} \times \dfrac{\cancel{12}^6}{1} = \dfrac{66}{1} = 66$

Answer. $5\dfrac{1}{2} \times 12 = 66$

Division of a fraction is based on the multiplication process. Dividing by a number is the same as multiplying by the **reciprocal** of that number. Examples of reciprocals are shown.

Number	Reciprocal
$\dfrac{3}{4}$	$\dfrac{4}{3}$
$\dfrac{1}{2}$	$\dfrac{2}{1}$
$8 = \dfrac{8}{1}$	$\dfrac{1}{8}$
$3\dfrac{1}{4} = \dfrac{13}{4}$	$\dfrac{4}{13}$
$2\dfrac{1}{2} = \dfrac{5}{2}$	$\dfrac{2}{5}$

> **RULE 1.9 Rule for Dividing Fractions**
>
> **Step 1.** Find the reciprocal of the divisor.
>
> **Step 2.** Multiply the dividend by the reciprocal of the divisor.
>
> **Step 3.** Reduce the quotient to lowest terms. Change any improper fraction to a mixed number.
>
> $$a \div b =$$
>
> Dividend → $a \times \dfrac{1}{b}$ ← Divisor ($b \neq 0$)
>
> $\uparrow$
> Reciprocal of divisor

EXAMPLE 1.18

(a) $\dfrac{3}{5} \div \dfrac{2}{4} =$

Step 1. The reciprocal of $\dfrac{2}{4}$ is $\dfrac{4}{2}$.

Step 2. $\dfrac{3}{5} \times \dfrac{4}{2} = \dfrac{12}{10} = 1\dfrac{2}{10} = 1\dfrac{1}{5}$

$\uparrow$
Multiply by the reciprocal of the divisor.

Answer. $\dfrac{3}{5} \div \dfrac{2}{4} = 1\dfrac{1}{5}$

(b) $\dfrac{4}{6} \div \dfrac{3}{9} =$

Step 1. The reciprocal of $\dfrac{3}{9}$ is $\dfrac{9}{3}$.

Step 2. $\dfrac{4}{6} \times \dfrac{9}{3} =$

$\dfrac{\cancel{4}^2}{\cancel{6}_{\cancel{2}_1}} \times \dfrac{\cancel{9}^{\cancel{3}^1}}{\cancel{3}_1} = \dfrac{2}{1} = 2$

1.3. Operations with Fractions and Mixed Numbers

Answer. $\dfrac{4}{6} \div \dfrac{3}{9} = 2$

RULE 1.10 Rule for Dividing Mixed Numbers

Step 1. Change each mixed number to an improper fraction.

Step 2. Find the reciprocal of the divisor.

Step 3. Multiply the dividend by the reciprocal of the divisor.

Step 4. Reduce the product. Change any improper fraction to a mixed number.

EXAMPLE 1.19

$3\dfrac{1}{5} \div 2\dfrac{1}{4} =$

Step 1. $\dfrac{16}{5} \div \dfrac{9}{4} =$

Step 2. The reciprocal of $\dfrac{9}{4}$ is $\dfrac{4}{9}$.

Step 3. $\dfrac{16}{5} \times \dfrac{4}{9} = \dfrac{64}{45} = 1\dfrac{19}{45}$

Answer. $3\dfrac{1}{5} \div 2\dfrac{1}{4} = 1\dfrac{19}{45}$

PRACTICE SET 1.3

Perform the indicated operations. Reduce all answers and change all improper fractions to mixed numbers.

1. $\dfrac{5}{8} + \dfrac{7}{8} =$

2. $\dfrac{3}{10} + \dfrac{7}{10} =$

3. $1\dfrac{4}{5} + 2\dfrac{3}{5} =$

4. $2\dfrac{9}{16} + 1\dfrac{13}{16} =$

5. $1\dfrac{5}{8} + 2\dfrac{5}{8} =$

6. $\dfrac{5}{12} - \dfrac{1}{12} =$

7. $\dfrac{13}{18} - \dfrac{4}{18} =$

8. $5\dfrac{5}{10} - 3\dfrac{3}{10} =$

9. $4\dfrac{5}{8} - 2\dfrac{3}{8} =$

10. $6\dfrac{8}{15} - 4\dfrac{7}{15} =$

Find the LCD. Perform the indicated operations. Reduce all answers to lowest terms. Change all improper fractions to mixed numbers.

11. $\dfrac{3}{18} + \dfrac{5}{24} =$

12. $\dfrac{1}{8} + \dfrac{2}{15} + \dfrac{1}{12} =$

13. $\dfrac{5}{16} - \dfrac{3}{10} =$

14. $\dfrac{5}{9} - \dfrac{4}{15} =$

15. $\dfrac{5}{9} - \dfrac{2}{10} + \dfrac{7}{30} =$

16. $7\dfrac{3}{8} + 2\dfrac{4}{5} =$

17. $62\dfrac{1}{2} + 16\dfrac{2}{3} =$

18. $7\dfrac{5}{10} - 2\dfrac{3}{8} =$

19. $6\dfrac{8}{15} - 4\dfrac{7}{12} =$

20. $14\dfrac{23}{60} - 5\dfrac{11}{12} =$

Perform the indicated operations. Reduce all answers to lowest terms. Change all improper fractions to mixed numbers.

21. $\dfrac{4}{9} \times \dfrac{3}{12} =$

22. $\dfrac{10}{25} \times \dfrac{10}{21} =$

23. $\dfrac{2}{3} \times \dfrac{12}{25} \times \dfrac{5}{8} =$

24. $1\dfrac{1}{3} \times 2\dfrac{1}{2} =$

25. $2\dfrac{2}{8} \times 3\dfrac{1}{3} =$

26. $\dfrac{10}{21} \div \dfrac{5}{7} =$

27. $\dfrac{3}{4} \div 2 =$

28. $18 \div \dfrac{1}{2} =$

29. $7\dfrac{1}{2} \div 3\dfrac{3}{4} =$

30. $5\dfrac{5}{6} \div 2\dfrac{4}{5} =$

1.4 CHAPTER REVIEW PROBLEMS

Write a fraction to express the portion of each figure that is shaded.

1.

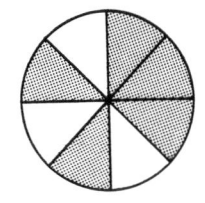

2.

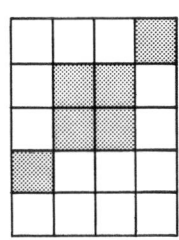

3.

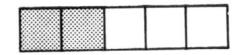

4.

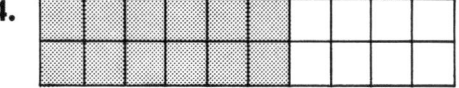

5. Write the fraction whose numerator is 6 and whose denominator is 10.

6. In the fraction $\frac{3}{5}$, name the denominator.

Change each of the following improper fractions to an equivalent mixed number.

7. $\frac{9}{2}$ **8.** $\frac{28}{11}$ **9.** $\frac{17}{3}$

10. $\frac{21}{5}$ **11.** $\frac{100}{25}$ **12.** $\frac{9}{5}$

13. $\frac{121}{10}$ **14.** $\frac{91}{8}$ **15.** $\frac{140}{11}$

16. $\frac{131}{20}$

Change each of the following mixed numbers to an equivalent improper fraction.

17. $1\frac{3}{4}$ **18.** $1\frac{4}{9}$ **19.** $5\frac{2}{5}$

20. $6\frac{1}{4}$ **21.** $3\frac{2}{3}$ **22.** $2\frac{7}{8}$

23. $4\frac{2}{10}$ **24.** $6\frac{2}{3}$ **25.** $8\frac{3}{4}$

26. $9\frac{4}{5}$

Change each of the following fractions to an equivalent fraction.

27. $\frac{1}{2} \times \frac{10}{10} =$

28. $\frac{5}{6} \times \frac{4}{4} =$

29. $\frac{7}{8} \times \frac{9}{9} =$

30. $\frac{2}{5} \times \frac{20}{20} =$

31. $\frac{7}{8} \times \frac{3}{3} =$

Reduce each of the following fractions to lowest terms.

32. $\frac{4}{6}$ **33.** $\frac{9}{12}$

34. $\frac{15}{18}$ **35.** $\frac{11}{15}$

36. $\frac{14}{35}$ **37.** $\frac{14}{16}$

38. $\frac{34}{38}$ **39.** $\frac{28}{49}$

40. $\frac{17}{51}$ **41.** $\frac{65}{75}$

Perform the indicated operations. Reduce all answers. Change all improper fractions to mixed numbers.

42. $\frac{2}{10} + \frac{6}{10} =$ **43.** $\frac{5}{8} - \frac{3}{8} =$

44. $\frac{3}{8} + \frac{5}{12} =$ **45.** $\frac{5}{9} - \frac{3}{8} =$

1.5. Chapter 1 Self Test

46. $\dfrac{5}{6} + \dfrac{3}{8} - \dfrac{7}{12} =$

47. $\dfrac{11}{16} + \dfrac{5}{6} - \dfrac{1}{2} =$

48. $2\dfrac{3}{8} + 1\dfrac{1}{4} =$

49. $7\dfrac{1}{3} + 5\dfrac{3}{5} =$

50. $3\dfrac{4}{7} - 1\dfrac{5}{8} =$

51. $9\dfrac{1}{4} - 5\dfrac{17}{32} =$

52. $\dfrac{2}{3} \times \dfrac{6}{10} =$

53. $\dfrac{8}{13} \times \dfrac{39}{40} \times \dfrac{5}{9} =$

54. $6\dfrac{7}{8} \times 1\dfrac{1}{5} =$

55. $3 \times 5\dfrac{3}{18} =$

56. $6\dfrac{1}{3} \times 2\dfrac{2}{5} \times 3\dfrac{3}{4} =$

57. $\dfrac{3}{4} \div \dfrac{1}{2} =$

58. $3 \div \dfrac{1}{3} =$

59. $3\dfrac{3}{4} \div \dfrac{5}{8} =$

60. $8\dfrac{2}{3} \div 3\dfrac{1}{4} =$

1.5 CHAPTER 1 SELF TEST

1.1 **1.**

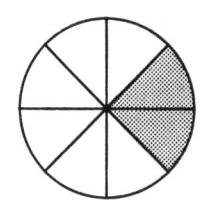

(a) Represent the fractional part that is shaded. _____

(b) Represent the fractional part that is not shaded. _____

1.2 **2.** Change each of the following improper fractions to an equivalent mixed number.

(a) $\dfrac{29}{4} =$ _____   (b) $\dfrac{105}{10} =$ _____

1.2 **3.** Change each of the following mixed fractions to an equivalent improper fraction.

(a) $5\dfrac{4}{5}$ _____   (b) $15\dfrac{1}{3}$ _____

1.2 **4.** Reduce each fraction to lowest terms.

(a) $\dfrac{75}{90} = $ _____   (b) $\dfrac{48}{84} = $ _____

1.2 **5.** Find the equivalent fraction for each given fraction.

(a) $\dfrac{5}{6} \times \dfrac{6}{6} = $ _____   (b) $\dfrac{2}{9} \times \dfrac{9}{9} = $ _____

1.3 **6.** Add and reduce each sum to lowest terms. Change any improper fraction to a mixed number.

(a) $\dfrac{5}{9} + \dfrac{7}{9} = $ _____   (b) $12\dfrac{4}{5} + 6\dfrac{2}{9} = $ _____

1.3 **7.** Subtract and reduce each difference to lowest terms.

(a) $\dfrac{5}{16} - \dfrac{3}{10} = $ _____   (b) $6\dfrac{7}{15} - 4\dfrac{6}{12} = $ _____

1.3 **8.** Multiply and reduce each product to lowest terms. Change any improper fraction to a mixed number.

(a) $\dfrac{4}{3} \times \dfrac{3}{10} = $ _____   (b) $3\dfrac{5}{7} \times 1\dfrac{3}{13} = $ _____

1.3 **9.** Divide and reduce each quotient to lowest terms. Change any improper fraction to a mixed number.

(a) $\dfrac{5}{8} \div \dfrac{4}{3} = $ _____   (b) $3\dfrac{3}{15} \div 2\dfrac{4}{5} = $ _____

1.3 **10.** The reciprocal of $\dfrac{5}{9} = $ _____

1.3 **11.** Find the LCD for $\dfrac{1}{4}, \dfrac{1}{9},$ and $\dfrac{1}{10}$ _____

1.1 **12.** If 7 equal parts of a figure are shaded, and there are 10 equal parts in the whole, write the fraction representing the unshaded parts.

_____

1.2 **13.** What fractional form of 1 was used to multiply the given fraction to get the equivalent fraction?

$\dfrac{2}{3} \times \dfrac{?}{?} = \dfrac{26}{39}$ _____

Summary of Chapter 1 Rules

1.3   **14.** $\dfrac{22}{7} \times \dfrac{7}{18} \times \dfrac{6}{77} =$ _____

1.2   **15.** Reduce to lowest terms. $\dfrac{4}{4} =$ _____

SUMMARY OF CHAPTER 1 RULES

RULE 1.1 Rule for Changing an Improper Fraction to a Mixed Number

Step 1. Divide the numerator by the denominator.

Step 2. Write this quotient followed by the fraction: $\dfrac{\text{remainder}}{\text{divisor}}$.

RULE 1.2 Rule for Changing a Mixed Number to an Improper Fraction

Step 1. Multiply the denominator by the whole number.

Step 2. Add the numerator to the product obtained in Step 1.

Step 3. Write the sum from Step 2 as the numerator in a fraction. The denominator is the denominator of the original fraction.

RULE 1.3 Rule for Reducing Fractions to Lowest Terms

Divide both the numerator and the denominator by the greatest common factor.

RULE 1.4 Rule for Adding or Subtracting Fractions with Common Denominators

Step 1. Add or subtract the numerators.

Step 2. Write the sum or the difference as the numerator of a fraction and the common denominator as the denominator.

Step 3. Reduce the fraction to lowest terms. Change all improper fractions to mixed numbers.

RULE 1.5 Rule for Finding the Least Common Denominator (LCD)

Step 1. Write the denominators in a horizontal line.

Step 2. Find a prime factor that divides exactly into at least two of the denominators. Write the quotients on the line below.

Step 3. Any denominator not divided exactly by the prime factor is brought down to the line below.

Step 4. Repeat this division step until no prime number divides at least two denominators on the quotient line.

Step 5. Multiply all the prime factors by all the numbers on the last quotient line.

RULE 1.6 Rule for Adding and Subtracting Fractions with Unlike Denominators

Step 1. Find the LCD.

Step 2. Convert each fraction to an equivalent fraction having the LCD as its denominator.

Step 3. Add or subtract the fractions.

Step 4. Reduce the answer to lowest terms. Change improper fractions to mixed numbers.

RULE 1.7 Rule for Multiplying Fractions

Step 1. Multiply numerators.

Step 2. Multiply denominators.

Step 3. Write the product of the numerators as the numerator of your answer and write the product of the denominators as the denominator of your answer.

Step 4. Reduce the fraction. Change the improper fractions to mixed numbers.

Summary of Chapter 1 Rules

RULE 1.8 Rule for Multiplying Mixed Numbers

Step 1. Change each mixed number to an equivalent improper fraction.

Step 2. Multiply the fractions. Cancel if possible.

Step 3. Reduce the fraction. Change any improper fraction to a mixed number.

RULE 1.9 Rule for Dividing Fractions

Step 1. Find the reciprocal of the divisor.

Step 2. Multiply the dividend by the reciprocal of the divisor.

Step 3. Reduce the quotient to lowest terms. Change any improper fraction to a mixed number.

$$a \div b =$$

Dividend → $a \times \dfrac{1}{b}$ ← Divisor ($b \neq 0$)

↑
Reciprocal of divisor

RULE 1.10 Rule for Dividing Mixed Numbers

Step 1. Change each mixed number to an improper fraction.

Step 2. Find the reciprocal of the divisor.

Step 3. Multiply the dividend by the reciprocal of the divisor.

Step 4. Reduce the product. Change any improper fraction to a mixed number.

2
Decimal Numbers

PRETEST

Chapter
Section

2.1   **1.** Write the word form for 4003.0065. _____

2.1   **2.** Write the decimal form for three hundred forty and three hundred forty hundred thousandths. _____

2.1   **3.** Name the place value of the underlined digit: 4176.01_3_4 _____

2.2   **4.** Round off 31.0975 to the nearest thousandth. _____

2.2   **5.** Which is greater: 1.90 or 1.090? _____

Perform the following operations.

2.3   **6.** 9.1 + 10 + 0.017 + 9.019 = _____

2.3   **7.** 91.07 − 63.753 = _____

2.3   **8.** 0.045 × 0.01 = _____

2.3   **9.** 16.4 ÷ 4 = _____

2.3   **10.** 122.5 ÷ 3.5 = _____

2.3   **11.** 354 ÷ 0.5 = _____

2.1. Reading and Writing Decimal Numbers

2.4   **12.** Change $\frac{2}{7}$ to a decimal number rounded to the nearest tenth. _____

2.4   **13.** Change $1\frac{1}{8}$ to its decimal equivalent. _____

2.4   **14.** A baby weighed 3.402 kilograms (kg) at birth. The baby now weighs 6.15 kg. How much weight in kg has the baby gained? _____

2.3   **15.** Yesterday a doctor delivered triplets at Huntington Memorial Hospital. The babies weighed 2 kg, 2.1 kg, and 3.01 kg. What was the sum weight of the triplets? _____

OBJECTIVES

After studying this chapter you should be able to

1. read and write decimals;
2. compare the size of decimals;
3. round decimal numbers to a given place value;
4. add, subtract, multiply, and divide decimal numbers;
5. change fractions and mixed numbers to decimal equivalents;
6. change decimals to fraction equivalents.

2.1 READING AND WRITING DECIMAL NUMBERS

A **decimal fraction** is a fraction whose denominator is a power of 10. A decimal fraction can be written as a decimal number by using a decimal point.

Some examples are:

Decimal fraction	*Decimal number*
$\frac{3}{10}$	0.3
$\frac{15}{100}$	0.15
$\frac{125}{1000}$	0.125

In studying decimal numbers, the place values must be memorized. Table 2–1 illustrates the place values of decimals. The decimal point is written be-

TABLE 2-1 PLACE VALUE CHART

Millions	Hundred thousands	Ten thousands	Thousands	Hundreds	Tens	Ones	Decimal point	Tenths	Hundredths	Thousandths	Ten thousandths	Hundred thousandths	Millionths
1,000,000	100,000	10,000	1,000	100	10	1	.	0.1	0.01	0.001	0.0001	0.00001	0.000001

tween the ones' place and the tenths' place. All the names of the place values to the right of the decimal point end in *ths*.

The value of each place is ten times the value of the place immediately to its right. For example:

> 0.1 is ten times 0.01
> 1 is ten times 0.1
> 10 is ten times 1
> 100 is ten times 10

EXAMPLE 2.1

Write the place value for the underlined digit.

Answer.

(a) 2<u>6</u>,540   Thousands

(b) <u>7</u>,920,435   Millions

(c) 0.00<u>5</u>   Thousandths

(d) 503.0<u>9</u>12   Hundredths

RULE 2.1   Rule for Reading a Decimal Number

Step 1. Read the number to the left of the decimal point as a whole number.

Step 2. Say *and* for the decimal point.

Step 3. Read the number to the right of the decimal point as a whole number.

Step 4. Then say the name of the place value of the rightmost digit of that number.

2.1. Reading and Writing Decimal Numbers

EXAMPLE 2.2

Write each of the following decimals in word form.

Answer.

(a) 5.06   Five and six hundredths
↑
Hundredths
place   Step 1   Step 2   Step 3   Step 4

(b) 2507.128   Two thousand, five hundred seven and one hundred twenty-eight thousandths
↑
Thousandths
place

(c) 0.6   Six tenths
↑
Tenths
place

RULE 2.2 Rule for Writing a Decimal Number Described in Words

Step 1. Write the whole number part. (If there is no whole number part, write 0 and a decimal point. Skip Step 2.)

Step 2. Write a decimal point for the word *and*.

Step 3. The last word(s) indicates the place value of the rightmost digit. Write the decimal part so as to give the rightmost digit the stated value.

EXAMPLE 2.3

Write each of the word forms in decimal form.

(a)   **Step 1**   **Step 2**   **Step 3**
         ↓   ↓   ↓
    Seventeen and six hundredths
                      ↑
       17.06   Place value of rightmost digit
        ↑
         The rightmost digit of the number must be written in the mentioned place value.

(b) Step 1 Step 2   Step 3
   ↓   ↓   ↓
   Four and seventeen thousandths

                    4.017
                      ↑
                    The rightmost digit of the number must
                    be written in the mentioned place value.

PRACTICE SET 2.1

Write each of the following numbers in word form. Name the place value of each underlined digit.

1. 5.0<u>1</u>5
2. 1<u>3</u>.5
3. 1<u>4</u>97.0900
4. 0.001<u>0</u>7
5. 9,<u>5</u>06,000.09

Write each of the following word forms of numbers in decimal form.

6. Sixty-two and five hundred twenty-five ten thousandths
7. Thirteen and two hundredths
8. One hundred thirty-seven hundred thousandths
9. Two thousand, twenty-five and six millionths
10. Nine million, fifty thousand, two and six thousandths

2.2 COMPARING AND ROUNDING OFF DECIMAL NUMBERS

The sizes of decimals can be compared by writing each of them with the same number of decimal places.

EXAMPLE 2.4

Which is the larger decimal number?

(a) 0.27 or 0.250

Since the largest number of decimal places to the right of the decimal point in either of the numbers is three, write each number with three decimal places. This can be done by adding zeros to the right of the decimal point.

$$0.250 = 0.250$$
$$0.27 = 0.270$$

2.2. Comparing and Rounding off Decimal Numbers

Now compare.

Answer. 0.270 is larger then 0.250.

(b) 0.110 or 0.99

Write 0.99 as 0.990.
Compare 0.990 with 0.110.

Answer. 0.990 is larger than 0.110.

EXAMPLE 2.5

Write each of the following decimals in descending order according to size.

$$3.1, 3.0501, 3.05, 3.107, 3.5$$

Rewrite each decimal as a number with four places to the right of the decimal point.

$$3.1 = 3.1000$$
$$3.0501 = 3.0501$$
$$3.05 = 3.0500$$
$$3.107 = 3.1070$$
$$3.5 = 3.5000$$

Compare each decimal.
Write in descending order:

$$3.5000, 3.1070, 3.1000, 3.0501, 3.0500$$

Answer. The original decimal numbers written in descending order are: 3.5, 3.107, 3.1, 3.0501, 3.05

Sometimes there is a need to round off decimal numbers to a given place value.

RULE 2.3 Rule for Rounding Off a Decimal Number to a Given Place Value

Step 1. Place an arrow under the digit of the given place value.

Step 2. Circle the digit immediately to the right of the digit with the arrow.

Step 3. If the circled digit is 5, 6, 7, 8, or 9, add 1 to the digit with the arrow. If the circled digit is 0, 1, 2, 3, or 4, the digit with the arrow remains unchanged.

Step 4. Discard all the digits to the right of the arrow and leave all the digits to the left of the arrow unchanged.

EXAMPLE 2.6

Round 0.00013 to the nearest ten thousandth.

Step 1. Draw an arrow under the 1, the digit in the ten-thousandths place.

0.00013
     ↑

Step 2. Circle the 3, the digit to the right of the arrow.

0.0001③
     ↑

Step 3. Since the circled digit is a 3, the digit above the arrow remains unchanged.

Step 4. Discard all digits to the right of the arrow. All digits to the left of the arrow remain unchanged.

0.0001

Answer. 0.00013 rounded off to the nearest ten thousandth is 0.0001.

EXAMPLE 2.7

Round 4.87654 to the nearest hundredth.

Step 1. Draw an arrow under 7, the digit in the hundredths place.

4.87654
   ↑

Step 2. Circle the 6, the digit to the right of the arrow.

4.87⑥54
   ↑

Step 3. Since the circled digit is a 6, add one to the digit with the arrow.

+1
4.87⑥54
   ↓
   8

Step 4. Discard all the digits to the right of the arrow. All digits to the left of the arrow remain unchanged.

+1
4.87⑥54 = 4.88
   ↓
   8

Answer. 4.87654 rounded to the nearest hundredth is 4.88.

2.2. Comparing and Rounding off Decimal Numbers

EXAMPLE 2.8

Round 9.96 to the nearest tenth.

Step 1. 9.96
 ↑

Step 2. 9.9⑥
 ↑
 +1
Step 3. 9.9⑥
 ↑
 +1
Step 4. 9.9⑥ The addition makes carrying necessary.
 ↓   9.9
 10.0 + .1
       ─────
       10.0

Answer. 9.96 rounded to the nearest tenth is 10.0.

PRACTICE SET 2.2

Which decimal number is larger?

1. 1.16 or 1.2

2. 0.99 or 0.909

3. 4.051 or 4.50

Write the following decimal numbers in descending order according to size.

4. 1.4, 1.401, 1.0440, 1.440

5. 0.2, 0.201, 0.020, 0.0222

Round off each of the following numbers to the indicated place value.

6. 2.817 (to the nearest tenth)

7. 4.499 (to the nearest hundredth)

8. 0.00155 (to the nearest ten thousandth)

9. 7.81 (to the nearest one)

10. 5654.1 (to the nearest one)

2.3 OPERATIONS WITH DECIMAL NUMBERS

Only digits with the same place values may be added to or subtracted from each other.

RULE 2.4 Rule for Adding and Subtracting Decimal Numbers

Step 1. Write the numbers in a vertical column with the decimal points lined up

Step 2. Add or subtract the numbers like whole numbers.

Step 3. Place the decimal point in the answer in the same position as the other decimal points.

EXAMPLE 2.9

Add or subtract as indicated.

(a) 7.5 + 0.077 + 80.75 + 267 =

```
  7.5        Step 1. Decimal points are lined up.
  0.077
 80.75       Step 2. Numbers are added.
267.
───────
355.327      Step 3. Decimal point in answer is written in the same posi-
                     tion as the other decimal points.
```

Answer.   7.5 + 0.077 + 80.75 + 267 = 355.327

(b) 12.87 − 4.3 =

Decimal points are written in a vertical column.

```
 12.87
− 4.3
──────
  8.57
```

Decimal point is in the same vertical column as the other decimal points.

Answer.   12.87 − 4.3 = 8.57

The multiplication of decimal numbers requires a different rule.

2.3. Operations with Decimal Numbers

> **RULE 2.5 Rule for Multiplying Decimal Numbers**
>
> **Step 1.** Multiply the two numbers as whole numbers.
>
> **Step 2.** Count the number of digits to the right of the decimal point in each of the two numbers being multiplied.
>
> **Step 3.** Place the decimal point in the product so that there are as many digits to the right of the decimal point as counted in Step 2.

EXAMPLE 2.10

Multiply:

(a) $2.564 \times 0.35 =$

Step 1. Multiply as whole numbers.

$2.564 \times 0.35 = 89740$

Step 2. Count the number of digits to the right of the decimal point in the two numbers being multiplied.

2.564 × 0.35

3 digits + 2 digits = 5 digits to the right of the decimal point

Step 3. Place the decimal point in the product so that there are 5 digits to the right of it.

$2.564 \times 0.35 = 0.89740$

Answer. $2.564 \times 0.35 = 0.89740$

(b) $0.56 \times 0.0049 =$

```
 0.56   ← 2 digits to the right of decimal point
 0.0049 ← 4 digits to the right of decimal point
 ──────
   504
   224
 ──────
 0.002744
```

Place the decimal point so that there are 6 places to the right of the decimal point. Zeros should be added if needed.

Answer. $0.56 \times 0.0049 = 0.002744$

There are two cases to consider in the division of decimal numbers. Both cases require careful positioning of the decimal point.

> **RULE 2.6 Case 1: Rule for Dividing a Decimal Number by a Whole Number**
>
> **Step 1.** Place the decimal point in the quotient directly above the decimal point in the dividend.
>
> **Step 2.** Divide the numbers as usual.

EXAMPLE 2.11

Divide as indicated.

(a) 26.52 ÷ 3 =
    ↑   ↑
    Dividend divisor

```
      8.84      Step 1. Place decimal point in quotient directly above the
   3)26.52              decimal point in the dividend.
     24
     ——
      2 5
      2 4
      ——
        12
        12      Step 2. Divide.
        ——
         0
```

Answer. 26.54 ÷ 3 = 8.84

(b) 225.68 ÷ 32 = (Round off quotient to the nearest tenth.)

```
        7.05     Step 1. Place decimal point in quotient directly above deci-
   32)225.68            mal point in the dividend.
      224
      ———
       16
       00       Step 2. Divide. Division must be carried out to the hun-
       ——              dredths place and then rounded off to the tenths
       168             place.
       160
       ———
         8
```

Answer. 225.68 ÷ 32 = 7.1 (Rounded to the nearest tenth)

2.3. Operations with Decimal Numbers   43

RULE 2.7   Case II: Rule for Dividing a Decimal Number by a Decimal Number

Step 1. Place an arrow to the right of the rightmost digit in the divisor.

Step 2. Count the number of places between the decimal point and the arrow.

Step 3. Place an arrow in the dividend the same number of places to the right of its decimal point as was counted in Step 2. Add zeros if needed.

Step 4. Place the decimal point in the quotient directly above the arrow in the dividend.

Step 5. Divide the numbers as though the divisor were a whole number.

EXAMPLE 2.12

Divide as indicated.

(a)   3.75 ÷ 2.5 =
       ↑   ↑
    Dividend Divisor

   Step 1. Place arrow to the right of rightmost digit in the divisor.

$$2.5\overline{)3.75}$$
       ↑

   Step 2. Count the number of places between the decimal point and the arrow.

$$2.5\overline{)3.75}$$
       ↑

   One place between arrow and the decimal point

   Step 3. Place arrow in dividend one place to the right of its decimal point.

$$2.5\overline{)3.75}$$
       ↑   ↑

   Step 4. Place decimal point in quotient directly above arrow in the dividend.

$$2.5\overline{)3.75}$$
       ↑   ↑

Step 5. Divide as though the divisor were a whole number.

$$\begin{array}{r} 1.5 \\ 2.5\overline{\smash{)}3.75} \\ \underline{\uparrow 25\uparrow} \\ 125 \\ \underline{125} \\ 0 \end{array}$$

Answer. $3.75 \div 2.5 = 1.5$

(b) $0.0926 \div 2.4 =$ Give quotient rounded off to the nearest thousandth.

$$\begin{array}{r} 0.0385 \\ 2.4\overline{\smash{)}0.09260} \\ \underline{\uparrow 72} \\ 206 \\ \underline{192} \\ 0140 \\ \underline{0120} \\ 20 \end{array}$$

— This zero was added to hold the place value above the 9.

One place

A zero was added so that division could be carried out to the ten thousandths place. Only then could the decimal be rounded off to the nearest thousandth.

Answer. $0.926 \div 2.4 = 0.039$ (Rounded off to the nearest thousandth)

PRACTICE SET 2.3

Perform the indicated operations.

1. $27.4 + 141 + 5.7 + 0.072 =$
2. $39 + 7.8 + 3.56 + 0.5 =$
3. $59.3 + 105 + 11 + 9.2 + 0.071 =$
4. $17.39 - 2.6 =$
5. $49.07 - 0.918 =$
6. $20 - 12.29 =$
7. $0.56 \times 0.049 =$
8. $7.8 \times 0.125 =$
9. $60.3 \times 0.508 =$
10. $43.75 \div 7 =$
11. $59.75 \div 18 =$ (Round quotient to the nearest hundredth.)

2.4. Converting Common Fractions and Mixed Numbers to Decimal Numbers

12. 1384.1 ÷ 56 = (Round quotient to the nearest tenth.)

13. 71.61 ÷ 2.1 =

14. 219.25 ÷ 0.046 = (Round quotient to the nearest one.)

15. 15.637 ÷ 2.35 = (Round quotient to the nearest hundredth.)

2.4 CONVERTING COMMON FRACTIONS AND MIXED NUMBERS TO DECIMAL NUMBERS; CHANGING DECIMALS TO FRACTIONS

If the numerator of a fraction is divided by its denominator and a decimal point is used, the quotient is an equivalent decimal number.

RULE 2.8 Rule for Changing a Fraction to a Decimal Number

Divide the numerator by the denominator. Supply a decimal point and zeros as needed.

EXAMPLE 2.13

Change each of the following fractions to an equivalent decimal number.

(a) $\frac{2}{5}$

$$\begin{array}{r} 0.4 \\ 5\overline{)2.0} \end{array}$$
↑
Supply a decimal point and a zero.

Answer. $\frac{2}{5} = 0.4$

(b) $\frac{2}{3}$ (Round to the nearest hundredth.)

$$\begin{array}{r} 0.666 \\ 3\overline{)2.000} \end{array}$$

Answer. $\frac{2}{3} = 0.67$ (Rounded to the nearest hundredth)

Mixed numbers may be treated like common fractions.

EXAMPLE 2.14

Change $4\frac{3}{16}$ to its decimal equivalent.

First, change $\frac{3}{16}$ to its decimal equivalent.

$$\begin{array}{r} 0.1875 \\ 16\overline{)3.0000} \end{array}$$

Then combine the whole number part with the decimal equivalent.

Answer. $4\frac{3}{16} = 4.1875$

A decimal can also be changed to its fraction equivalent.

RULE 2.9 Rule for Changing a Decimal to a Fraction

Step 1. Write the place value of the rightmost digit in fractional form.

Step 2. Replace the numerator of this fraction with the original decimal number minus its decimal point.

Step 3. Reduce the fraction to lowest terms.

EXAMPLE 2.15

Change .44 to a fraction in lowest terms.

Step 1. Write the place value of the rightmost digit in fractional form.

0.44 Rightmost digit is in hundredths place.

One hundredth written as a fraction is $\frac{1}{100}$.

Step 2. Replace the numerator of this fraction with the original decimal number, 0.44, minus its decimal point.

$$\frac{1}{100} \Rightarrow \frac{44}{100}$$

Step 3. Reduce $\frac{44}{100}$ to lowest terms.

$$\frac{44}{100} = \frac{11}{25}$$

Answer. $0.44 = \frac{11}{25}$

PRACTICE SET 2.4

Change each of the given fractions and mixed numbers to its decimal equivalent.

1. $\frac{7}{8}$
2. $\frac{3}{5}$
3. $9\frac{3}{4}$
4. $\frac{5}{9}$ (Round off to the nearest hundredth.)
5. $1\frac{3}{7}$ (Round off to the nearest thousandth.)

Change each decimal to a fraction in lowest terms.

6. 0.15
7. 0.375
8. 0.125
9. 0.8
10. 0.0625

2.5 CHAPTER 2 REVIEW PROBLEMS

Write the place value of the underlined digit.

1. 7.01<u>6</u>1
2. 13.<u>7</u>19
3. <u>9</u>,753.16
4. 317.1694<u>5</u>
5. <u>3</u>,507,611.1

Write each of the following decimal numbers in word form.

6. 9607.05
7. 13.0065
8. 0.00091
9. 3.000500
10. 1004007.9

Write each of the following word form numbers in decimal form.

11. Thirty-seven thousandths
12. Three and one hundred fifteen millionths
13. Two thousand, forty-one and six hundredths
14. One million, two hundred thousand and five tenths
15. Twenty-seven thousand, three and four ten thousandths

Write the following decimal numbers in descending order according to size.

16. 3.33, 3.0330, 3.333, 3.0033

17. 1.01, 1.001, 1.100, 1.011

18. 10.9, 10.99, 10.099, 10.999

Round off each of the following decimal numbers to the indicated place value.

19. 16.0913 (to the nearest tenth)

20. 94.1 (to the nearest ten)

21. 356.555 (to the nearest hundredth)

22. 413.916 (to the nearest one)

23. 0.05119 (to the nearest thousandth)

24. 516,914.0917 (to the nearest thousandth)

25. 1.00141 (to the nearest ten-thousandth)

Perform the operations as indicated.

26. 18.54 + 22.8 + 4 + 0.071 =

27. 515 + 0.017 + 2.1 + 3 =

28. 0.29 + 1.3 + 95 + 1.111 =

29. 14.83 − 5.6 =

30. 500 − 3.16 =

31. 0.517 − 0.21 =

32. 0.01 × 2.87 =

33. 0.96 × 100 =

34. 0.0268 × 0.0036 =

35. 265.81 ÷ 6 = (Round off the quotient to the nearest hundredth.)

36. 5.75 ÷ 0.63 = (Round off the quotient to the nearest hundredth.)

37. 514 ÷ 0.23 = (Round off the quotient to the nearest tenth.)

Change each of the following fractions or mixed numbers to its decimal equivalent.

38. $\dfrac{1}{8}$

39. $\dfrac{7}{6}$ (to the nearest hundredth)

40. $2\dfrac{1}{12}$ (to the nearest thousandth)

2.6. Chapter 2 Self-Test

Solve the following word problems.

41. Ms. Yamato has been taking 0.6 grams (g) of aspirin daily. If she has taken a total of 12.6 g of aspirin, how many days has she been taking this medicine?

42. Mrs. Sullivan has been placed on a special diet of 1.25 g of salt per day. How many grams of salt will Mrs. Sullivan consume in 120 days?

43. A patient suffering from a urinary infection is given 0.15 g of sulfisoxazole daily. If the patient must take this medicine for 10.5 days, how many grams of sulfisoxazole will she consume?

44. A doctor asks you to administer 1.2 milligrams (mg) of a drug four times daily. What is the total number of mg that you will administer in a week?

45. A child with a body surface of 1.07 square meters (m^2) is to be given 2.5 mg Valium for every m^2 of body surface. How many milligrams of Valium should be administered?

46. A patient is to be administered 2 ounces (oz) of medicine. What fractional part of a glass is this? (1 glass equals 8 oz.)

47. A patient is to be administered $3\frac{6}{7}$ oz of medicine. Write the decimal equivalent of this amount rounded off to the nearest hundredth.

2.6 CHAPTER 2 SELF TEST

2.1   **1.** Write the word form for each of the following decimals.
     (a) 27.0150 _____
     (b) 1030.001 _____

2.1   **2.** Write each of the following word form numbers in decimal form.
     (a) Twenty-seven thousand and five hundredths _____
     (b) Five hundred fourteen hundred thousandths _____

2.1   **3.** Name the place value of the underlined digit.
     (a) 47.10159$\underline{6}$ _____
     (b) 1$\underline{5}$43.718 _____

2.2   **4.** Round off each of the following decimal numbers to the indicated place value.
     (a) 1.019 (to the nearest hundredth) _____
     (b) 1944.09 (to the nearest tenth) _____
     (c) 54.55 (to the nearest tenth) _____

Perform the indicated operations.

2.3   **5.** $90 + 1.15 + 0.076 + 1.1 =$ _____

2.3   **6.** $514.1 - 13.06 =$ _____

2.3   **7.** $4.01 \times .011 =$ _____

2.3   **8.** $520.2 \div 41 =$ (Round off the quotient to the nearest one.) _____

2.3   **9.** $0.0187 \div .16 =$ (Round off the quotient to the nearest hundredth.) _____

2.3   **10.** $5 \div 0.22 =$ (Round off the quotient to the nearest tenth.) _____

2.4   **11.** Change $2\frac{5}{8}$ to its decimal equivalent. _____

2.4   **12.** Change $\frac{2}{3}$ to its decimal equivalent rounded to the nearest hundredth. _____

2.2   **13.** Which is the greater of the two decimal numbers? 4.100 or 4.0100 _____

2.3   **14.** Blood sample A contains a barbiturate level of 1.5 mg per 100 milliliters (mL) of blood. Blood sample B contains 1.47 mg per 100 mL of blood. What is the difference in the barbiturate levels? _____

2.3   **15.** A doctor prescribes 0.25 mg of reserpine twice daily for a patient with high blood pressure. The patient is to take this medication for 2 weeks. How many mg will she have taken at the end of the 2 weeks? _____

SUMMARY OF CHAPTER 2 RULES

> **RULE 2.1 Rule for Reading a Decimal Number**
>
> **Step 1.** Read the number to the left of the decimal point as a whole number.
> **Step 2.** Say *and* for the decimal point.
> **Step 3.** Read the number to the right of the decimal point as a whole number.
> **Step 4.** Then say the name of the place value of the rightmost digit of that number.

Summary of Chapter 2 Rules

> **RULE 2.2 Rule for Writing a Decimal Number Described in Words**
>
> **Step 1.** Write the whole number part. (If there is no whole number part, write 0 and a decimal point. Skip Step 2.)
> **Step 2.** Write a decimal point for the word *and*.
> **Step 3.** The last word(s) indicates the place value of the rightmost digit. Write the decimal part so as to give the rightmost digit the stated value.

> **RULE 2.3 Rule for Rounding Off a Decimal Number to a Given Place Value**
>
> **Step 1.** Place an arrow under the digit of the given place value.
> **Step 2.** Circle the digit immediately to the right of the digit with the arrow.
> **Step 3.** If the circled digit is 5, 6, 7, 8, or 9, add 1 to the digit with the arrow. If the circled digit is 0, 1, 2, 3, or 4, the digit with the arrow remains unchanged.
> **Step 4.** Discard all the digits to the right of the arrow and leave all the digits to the left of the arrow unchanged.

> **RULE 2.4 Rule for Adding and Subtracting Decimal Numbers**
>
> **Step 1.** Write the numbers in a vertical column with the decimal points lined up.
> **Step 2.** Add or subtract the numbers like whole numbers.
> **Step 3.** Place the decimal point in the answer in the same position as the other decimal points.

> **RULE 2.5 Rule for Multiplying Decimal Numbers**
>
> **Step 1.** Multiply the two numbers as whole numbers.
> **Step 2.** Count the number of digits to the right of the decimal point in each of the two numbers being multiplied.
> **Step 3.** Place the decimal point in the product so that there are as many digits to the right of the decimal point as counted in Step 2.

> **RULE 2.6 Case I: Rule for Dividing a Decimal Number by a Whole Number**
>
> **Step 1.** Place the decimal point in the quotient directly above the decimal point in the dividend.
>
> **Step 2.** Divide the numbers as usual.

> **RULE 2.7 Case II: Rule for Dividing a Decimal Number by a Decimal Number**
>
> **Step 1.** Place an arrow to the right of the rightmost digit in the divisor.
>
> **Step 2.** Count the number of places between the decimal point and the arrow.
>
> **Step 3.** Place an arrow in the dividend the same number of places to the right of its decimal point as was counted in Step 2. Add zeros if needed.
>
> **Step 4.** Place the decimal point in the quotient directly above the arrow in the dividend.
>
> **Step 5.** Divide the numbers as though the divisor were a whole number.

> **RULE 2.8 Rule for Changing a Fraction to a Decimal Number**
>
> Divide the numerator by the denominator. Supply a decimal point and zeros as needed.

> **RULE 2.9 Rule for Changing a Decimal to a Fraction**
>
> **Step 1.** Write the place value of the rightmost digit in fractional form.
>
> **Step 2.** Replace the numerator of this fraction with the original decimal number minus its decimal point.
>
> **Step 3.** Reduce the fraction to lowest terms.

3
Ratios, Proportions, and Percents

PRETEST

Chapter
Section

3.1   **1.** Write the following comparison in both colon and fractional form: 0.3 to 100 _____

3.2   **2.** Solve for x: $\dfrac{35}{x} = \dfrac{42}{56}$ _____

3.2   **3.** Solve for x: $\dfrac{0.05}{100} = \dfrac{0.025}{x}$ _____

3.3   **4.** Change 3.85% to its equivalent decimal form. _____

3.3   **5.** Change 0.3 to its equivalent percent form. _____

3.4   **6.** What number is 38% of 16? _____

3.4   **7.** 4.6% of what number is 11.5? _____

3.2   **8.** If a doctor orders 3 liters (L) of isotonic sodium chloride to be administered to a patient over a period of 18 hr, how many L will the patient have received in 48 hr? _____

3.2   **9.** A doctor prescribes 15 mg of Dimetane per m^2 for a patient with a body surface of 0.92 m^2. How many mg should be administered?

                _____

3.4   **10.** Herpes encephalitis has a death rate of about 70%. If 250 persons catch this particular viral infection, how many are expected to die?

                _____

OBJECTIVES

After studying this chapter, you will be able to

1. read and solve ratios and proportions;
2. solve and check a proportion;
3. convert percents to equivalent decimal numbers and decimal numbers to equivalent percent forms;
4. solve percent problems.

3.1 RATIOS AND PROPORTIONS

A **ratio** compares two numbers. For example, if the weights of two persons are compared, one weighing 120 pounds (lb) and another weighing 110 lb, the ratio would be 120 lb to 110 lb. This comparison can be written either using a colon or as a fraction. Both the colon and the fraction bar come from the division symbol ($\div$). The comparison of the two weights is:

$$120 : 110 \leftarrow \text{Colon form}$$

or

$$\frac{120}{110} \leftarrow \text{Fractional form}$$

EXAMPLE 3.1

Write the comparison of 3 to 4 in colon form and in fractional form.

	Colon form	*Fractional form*
	3 : 4	$\frac{3}{4}$
Read:	The ratio of three to four	Three fourths

3.1. Ratios and Proportions

EXAMPLE 3.2

Write the ratio of $2\frac{1}{2}$ to 1 in colon form and in fractional form.

Colon form	Fractional form
$2\frac{1}{2} : 1$	$\dfrac{2\frac{1}{2}}{1}$

In general a **ratio** can be defined as the comparison of two numbers, a and b ($b \neq 0$). This comparison can be written in either a colon form, $a : b$, or a fractional form, $\dfrac{a}{b}$ ($b \neq 0$).

EXAMPLE 3.3

There are 12 inches (in.) in 1 foot (ft). Write this in colon form and in fractional form.

Colon form	Fractional form
12 in. : 1 ft	$\dfrac{12 \text{ in.}}{1 \text{ ft}}$
or	or
1 ft : 12 in.	$\dfrac{1 \text{ ft}}{12 \text{ in.}}$

EXAMPLE 3.4

1 oz of solution contains 5 g drug. Write this in colon form and in fractional form.

Colon form	Fractional form
1 oz : 5 g	$\dfrac{1 \text{ oz}}{5 \text{ g}}$
or	or
5 g : 1 oz	$\dfrac{5 \text{ g}}{1 \text{ oz}}$

EXAMPLE 3.5

(a) A doctor's order reads, "Administer 5 L dextrose solution over a period of 24 hr." Write this in fractional form.

$$\frac{5 \text{ L dextrose}}{24 \text{ hours}}$$

(b) A doctor's order reads, "Administer 0.5 g drug per kg body mass." Write this in fractional form.

$$\frac{0.5 \text{ g}}{1 \text{ kg}}$$

A **proportion** is a statement that two ratios are equal. It can be thought of as an equation of two ratios. Here is an example of a proportion:

$$2 : 3 = 4 : 6 \quad \text{or} \quad \frac{2}{3} = \frac{4}{6}$$

The proportion on the left is read, "2 is to 3 as 4 is to 6." The proportion on the right may be read either as two ratios or two fractions: "2 is to 3 as 4 is to 6" or "two-thirds equals four-sixths."

The following are some rules applicable to a proportion.

RULE 3.1 Cross Products Rule

If two fractions are equivalent, their cross products are equal.

RULE 3.2 Cross Product Equality Rule

If the cross products of two fractions in a proportion are equal, then the fractions are equivalent. The proportion is true.

In the proportion $\frac{3}{4} = \frac{6}{8}$, the cross products are:

$$\frac{3}{4} \times \frac{6}{8}$$

$$3 \times 8 = 6 \times 4$$

$$24 = 24$$

The cross products are equal.

3.1. Ratios and Proportions

EXAMPLE 3.6

Show that the following fractions are equivalent by using the cross products rule.

(a) $\frac{1}{2} = \frac{4}{8} \Rightarrow \frac{1}{2} \times \frac{4}{8}$

$1 \times 8 = 4 \times 2$

$8 = 8 \quad$ Cross products are equal.

(b) $\frac{2}{3} = \frac{16}{24} \Rightarrow \frac{2}{3} \times \frac{16}{24}$

$2 \times 24 = 16 \times 3$

$48 = 48 \quad$ Cross products are equal.

EXAMPLE 3.7

Check to see if each proportion is true or false by using the cross products equality rule.

(a) $\frac{3}{4} \stackrel{?}{=} \frac{9}{12} \quad$ Does $3 \times 12 = 9 \times 4$?

$36 = 36$

The proportion is true; the fractions are equivalent.

(b) $\frac{2\frac{1}{3}}{7} \stackrel{?}{=} \frac{5}{15} \quad$ Does $2\frac{1}{3} \times 15 = 5 \times 7$?

$\frac{7}{3} \times 15 = 5 \times 7$

$35 = 35$

The proportion is true.

PRACTICE SET 3.1

Write each of the following numbers in colon form and in fractional form.

1. 10 to 12

2. $3\frac{1}{2}$ to 1

3. 10 mg per lb

4. 8 oz in 1 glass

5. 45 mL of Milk of Magnesia every 12 hr

Indicate if the following proportions are true or false.

6. $\dfrac{5}{7} \stackrel{?}{=} \dfrac{65}{91}$

7. $\dfrac{7}{2\frac{1}{2}} \stackrel{?}{=} \dfrac{14}{5}$

8. $\dfrac{18}{30} \stackrel{?}{=} \dfrac{1\frac{4}{5}}{2.5}$

9. $\dfrac{4.3}{5} \stackrel{?}{=} \dfrac{6.88}{8}$

10. $\dfrac{3.14}{4} \stackrel{?}{=} \dfrac{1.57}{2}$

3.2 SOLVING PROPORTIONS

A proportion can be written in the general form, $\dfrac{a}{b} = \dfrac{c}{d}$ where a, b, c, and d are called the **terms of proportion**. Neither b nor d can equal zero. Using these terms, the cross product rule can now be written in the following form:

$$a \times d = c \times b$$

There are other rules, called the **rules of equality**, that should be learned before proportions can be solved.

RULE 3.3 Rule of Equality for Addition

If the same number is added to each member of an equality, the sums are equal.

If $a = b$, then $a + c = b + c$

In Example 3.8, x is used to denote an unknown number.

3.2. Solving Proportions

EXAMPLE 3.8

(a) If $\quad x - 3 = 4$

then
$$\begin{array}{r} x - 3 = 4 \\ + 3 = +3 \\ \hline x + 0 = 7 \\ x = 7 \end{array}$$

3 was added to each member of the equality.

(b) If $\quad x - 2 = 10$

then
$$\begin{array}{r} x - 2 = 10 \\ + 2 = +2 \\ \hline x + 0 = 12 \\ x = 12 \end{array}$$

2 was added to each member of the equality.

RULE 3.4 Rule of Equality for Subtraction

If the same number is subtracted from each member of an equality, the differences are equal.

If $a = b$, then $a - c = b - c$

EXAMPLE 3.9

(a) If $\quad x + 1 = 6$

then
$$\begin{array}{r} x + 1 = 6 \\ - 1 = -1 \\ \hline x + 0 = 5 \\ x = 5 \end{array}$$

1 was subtracted from each member of the equality.

(b) If $\quad x + 6 = 12$

then
$$\begin{array}{r} x + 6 = 12 \\ - 6 = -6 \\ \hline x + 0 = 6 \\ x = 6 \end{array}$$

6 was subtracted from each member of the equality.

> **RULE 3.5 Rule of Equality for Multiplication**
>
> If each member of an equality is multiplied by the same number, the products are equal.
>
> If $a = b$, then $ac = bc$

EXAMPLE 3.10

(a) If $\dfrac{x}{2} = 6$

then $\left(\dfrac{2}{1}\right)\dfrac{x}{2} = \left(\dfrac{2}{1}\right)6$

$x = 12$

(Note that the parentheses indicate multiplication. Also, when a number and a letter are written together such as $5x$, multiplication is implied.)

Each member of the equality was multiplied by $\dfrac{2}{1}$.

(b) If $\dfrac{x}{4} = 3$

then $\left(\dfrac{4}{1}\right)\dfrac{x}{4} = \left(\dfrac{4}{1}\right)3$

$x = 12$

Each member of the equality was multiplied by $\dfrac{4}{1}$.

> **RULE 3.6 Rule of Equality for Division**
>
> If each member of an equality is divided by the same number (zero excluded), the quotients are equal.
>
> If $a = b$ and $c \neq 0$, then $\dfrac{a}{c} = \dfrac{b}{c}$.

EXAMPLE 3.11

(a) If $3x = 24$

then $\dfrac{3x}{3} = \dfrac{24}{3}$

$x = 8$

Each member of the equality was divided by 3.

3.2. Solving Proportions

(b) If $5x = 30$

then $\dfrac{5x}{5} = \dfrac{30}{5}$

$x = 6$

Each member of the equality was divided by 5.

As shown in the preceding example, if one term of a proportion is unknown, this term is represented by a letter, usually x. The proportion is solved when a value is found for this unknown quantity.

RULE 3.7 Rule for Solving a Proportion

Step 1. Write the cross products in equation form.

Step 2. Divide each member by the number that multiplies the unknown letter. (Use the rule of equality for division.)

Step 3. Simplify the equation.

EXAMPLE 3.12

Solve for x: $\dfrac{3}{7} = \dfrac{x}{21}$

Step 1. Write the cross products in equation form.

$$7x = (3)(21)$$

Step 2. Divide each product by the number 7.

$$\dfrac{7x}{7} = \dfrac{(3)(21)}{7}$$

Step 3.

$$\dfrac{\cancel{7}x}{\cancel{7}} = \dfrac{(3)(\cancel{21}^3)}{\cancel{7}}$$

$$x = (3)(3)$$

$$x = 9$$

The solution of a proportion can be checked by replacing the value of x in the proportion and using the cross products rule.

$$\frac{3}{7} = \frac{9}{21} \quad \leftarrow \text{Value for } x$$

$$(3)(21) = (9)(7)$$

$$63 = 63 \quad \text{Since the cross products are equal, the proportion is true. The solution is correct.}$$

EXAMPLE 3.13

Solve for x: $\dfrac{4}{5} = \dfrac{3}{x}$ Check

Step 1. $4x = (3)(5)$ Cross products

Step 2. $\dfrac{4x}{4} = \dfrac{(3)(5)}{4}$ Use rule of equality for division

Step 3. $\dfrac{\cancel{4}x}{\underset{1}{\cancel{4}}} = \dfrac{(3)(5)}{4}$

$$x = \frac{15}{4} = 3\frac{3}{4}$$

Check. $\dfrac{4}{5} = \dfrac{3}{3\dfrac{3}{4}}$

$$(4)\left(3\frac{3}{4}\right) = (3)(5)$$

$$(4)\left(3\frac{3}{4}\right) = (3)(5)$$

$$15 = 15 \quad \text{The proportion is true; the solution is correct.}$$

EXAMPLE 3.14

Solve and check the proportion.

$$\frac{x}{3\frac{1}{2}} = \frac{8}{14}$$

3.2. Solving Proportions

Step 1. $\qquad 14x = (8)\left(3\dfrac{1}{2}\right) \qquad$ Cross products

Step 2. $\qquad \dfrac{14x}{14} = \dfrac{(8)\left(3\dfrac{1}{2}\right)}{14} \qquad$ Use rule of equality for division

Step 3. $\qquad x = 2$

Check. $\qquad \dfrac{2}{3\dfrac{1}{2}} = \dfrac{8}{14}$

$$(2)(14) = (8)\left(3\dfrac{1}{2}\right)$$
$$28 = 28 \qquad \text{The proportion is true; the solution is correct.}$$

EXAMPLE 3.15

Solve and check the proportion.

$$\dfrac{2.2}{x} = \dfrac{8.8}{5}$$

Step 1. $\qquad 8.8x = (2.2)(5)$

Step 2. $\qquad \dfrac{8.8x}{8.8} = \dfrac{(2.2)(5)}{8.8}$

Step 3. $\qquad x = 1.25$

Check. $\qquad \dfrac{(2.2)}{1.25} = \dfrac{8.8}{5}$

$$(2.2)(5) = (8.8)(1.25)$$
$$11 = 11 \qquad \text{The proportion is true; the solution is correct.}$$

EXAMPLE 3.16

Solve and check the proportion.

$$\dfrac{3\dfrac{1}{2}}{x} = \dfrac{4.2}{8}$$

$$4.2x = \left(3\frac{1}{2}\right)(8)$$

$$\frac{4.2x}{4.2} = \frac{\left(3\frac{1}{2}\right)(8)}{4.2}$$

$$x = 6.7 \quad \text{(Rounded to the nearest tenth)}$$

Check.
$$\frac{3\frac{1}{2}}{6.7} = \frac{4.2}{8}$$

$$\left(3\frac{1}{2}\right)(8) = (4.2)(6.7)$$

$$28 \approx 28.14$$

This is not absolutely exact since 6.66 was rounded off to 6.7. Rounded-off values will sometimes produce a very minor discrepancy. ($\approx$ means "approximately.")

Ratios and proportions can be used to solve most medication problems. In dealing with word problems, first translate the given information into a proportion; then solve the proportion. Write labels for each term of the proportion. The labels in the numerators should match, as should the labels in the denominators.

EXAMPLE 3.17

A doctor's order reads, "Administer 0.9 g chloral hydrate every 48 hr." How many g should be administered in five days?

Information from problem:
Change 48 hr to 2 days, so that the labels will match in the denominators →

$$\frac{0.9 \text{ g}}{2 \text{ days}} = \frac{x \text{ g}}{5 \text{ days}} \quad \leftarrow \text{Like labels in numerators}$$

$$2x = (0.9)(5)$$

Answer. $x = 2.25$ g chloral hydrate

Check. $\dfrac{0.9}{2} = \dfrac{2.25}{5}$

$$(0.9)(5) = (2.25)(2)$$
$$4.5 = 4.5$$

3.2. Solving Proportions

EXAMPLE 3.18

Order: 0.3 g theophylline per m^2 body surface. How much theophylline should be administered to a patient with 1.3 m^2 body surface?

Information from problem:
$$\frac{0.3 \text{ g}}{1 \text{ m}^2} = \frac{x \text{ g}}{1.3 \text{ m}^2}$$

$$1x = (0.3)(1.3)$$

Answer. $x = 0.39$ g theophylline

Check.
$$\frac{0.3}{1} = \frac{0.39}{1.3}$$

$$(0.3)(1.3) = (0.39)(1)$$

$$0.39 = 0.39$$

There is a basic medication rule that makes use of the proportion.

RULE 3.8 Medication Rule

Ratio for Medication on Hand = Ratio for Desired Medication
(MOH)   (DM)

The medication on hand (MOH) is defined as the drug available in the supply room or from the pharmacy. The desired medication (DM) is the amount of drug prescribed by the physician to be administered to the patient.

EXAMPLE 3.19

60 mg of Tylenol is prescribed for a patient by the physician. If Tylenol elixir is available as 120 mg per 5 mL, how many mL should be administered to the patient?

Use the rule: MOH = DM
                 ↓   ↓
$$\frac{120 \text{ mg}}{5 \text{ mL}} = \frac{60 \text{ mg}}{x \text{ mL}}$$

$$120x = (60)(5)$$

$$120x = 300$$

$$\frac{120x}{120} = \frac{300}{120}$$

$$x = 2\frac{1}{2}$$

Answer. Administer $2\frac{1}{2}$ mL of Tylenol elixir.

PRACTICE SET 3.2

Solve and check each proportion.

1. $\dfrac{5}{9} = \dfrac{x}{117}$

2. $\dfrac{3}{7} = \dfrac{x}{91}$

3. $\dfrac{9}{x} = \dfrac{27}{100}$

4. $\dfrac{14}{x} = \dfrac{27}{100}$

5. $\dfrac{5}{2\frac{1}{2}} = \dfrac{12}{x}$

6. An injection of 4 mg of Valium has been prescribed for a patient suffering from muscle spasms. An ampule of Valium labeled 5 mg/mL is on hand. How many mL should be injected?

7. 5 mg of morphine sulfate have been prescribed for a patient suffering severe pain. If 15 mg/mL morphine sulfate are on hand, how many mL should be administered?

3.3 CONVERTING A PERCENT TO AN EQUIVALENT DECIMAL FORM AND A DECIMAL FORM TO AN EQUIVALENT PERCENT FORM

A **percent** is a ratio that compares a number to 100. A percent can be thought of as the number of parts per 100; that is, it can be a fraction whose denominator is 100.

$$45\% = \dfrac{45}{100} \qquad \dfrac{15}{100} = 15\% \qquad 10\% = \dfrac{10}{100} \qquad \dfrac{95}{100} = 95\%$$

3.3. Converting a Percent to an Equivalent Decimal Form

In general, it can be said that

$$N\% = \frac{N}{100} \quad \text{(The meaning of percent ratio)}$$

$$\frac{N}{100} = N \div 100$$

$$N \div 100 = N \times \frac{1}{100}$$

or

$$N \div 100 = N \times 0.01$$

This last statement will be used as a rule to change a percent to its equivalent decimal form.

> **RULE 3.9 Rule for Converting a Percent to Its Equivalent Decimal Form**
>
> To change from a percent to a decimal form, multiply by .01; that is, move the decimal point two places to the left.

EXAMPLE 3.20

Change each of the following percents to its equivalent decimal form.

(a) $15\% = 15 \times 0.01 = 0.15$

(b) $3.5\% = 3.5 \times 0.01 = 0.035$

(c) $\frac{3}{4}\% = \frac{3}{4} \times 0.01$

$= 0.75 \times 0.01 = 0.0075$

PRACTICE SET 3.3

Convert each of the following percents to its equivalent decimal form.

1. 37%
2. 82%
3. 400%
4. $\frac{1}{2}\%$

5. $12\frac{3}{4}\%$
6. $62\frac{1}{2}\%$
7. 0.8%
8. 38.6%
9. 0.27%
10. 0.08%
11. A bottle of potassium permanganate from the pharmacy is labeled 0.05% solution. Write this percent in its equivalent decimal form.
12. A doctor prescribed betamethasone benzoate for a patient. The label reads 0.025%. Write this percent in its equivalent decimal form.
13. A 75% solution of potassium iodide is available in a 50 cubic centimeter (cc) vial. Write this percent in its equivalent decimal form.

3.4 THE PERCENT PROPORTION

A basic percent proportion can be used to solve percent problems. Before percent problems can be solved, however, the percent statement must be investigated. A percent statement can be broken down into three categories: the percent, the whole, and the part.

$$\text{Percent} \Rightarrow \text{The number with the \%}$$
$$\text{Whole} \Rightarrow \text{Represents the entire amount}$$
$$\text{Part} \Rightarrow \text{Part of the whole}$$

EXAMPLE 3.21

Identify the three categories of the following percent questions.

(a) What is 15% of 200?
    ↑   ↑   ↑
  Part Percent Whole

(b) 150 is what percent of 600?
  ↑   ↑   ↑
  Part   Percent Whole

(c) 8 is 25% of what?
  ↑   ↑   ↑
  Part Percent Whole

Once the three categories of a percent statement have been identified, the percent, whole, and part can be put into a **percent proportion.**

3.4. The Percent Proportion

$$\text{Percent proportion} \Rightarrow \frac{\text{Percent}}{100} = \frac{\text{Part}}{\text{Whole}}$$

If one of these categories is unknown, the unknown quantity may be represented by the letter x.

EXAMPLE 3.22

Identify the percent, whole, and part in the following percent questions. Set them up in a percent proportion.

(a) 40% of 85 is what number?
     ↑   ↑   ↑
  Percent Whole   Part

  Percent proportion: Percent → $\frac{40}{100} = \frac{x}{85}$ ← Part
  ← Whole

(b) 8 is what % of 40?
     ↑   ↑   ↑
   Part Percent Whole

  Percent proportion: Percent → $\frac{x}{100} = \frac{8}{40}$ ← Part
  ← Whole

(c) 46 is 30% of what number?
     ↑   ↑   ↑
   Part Percent   Whole

  Percent proportion: Percent → $\frac{30}{100} = \frac{46}{x}$ ← Part
  ← Whole

RULE 3.10 Rule for Solving a Percent Proportion

Step 1. Identify the three categories of the percent statement: the percent, the whole, and the part.

Step 2. Set the percent, whole, and part into the percent proportion:
$$\frac{\text{percent}}{100} = \frac{\text{part}}{\text{whole}}$$
Represent the unknown quantity by x.

Step 3. Solve the proportion for the unknown quantity x.

Step 4. Check the solution.

EXAMPLE 3.23

Solve each of the following percent problems. Check the solution.

(a) What is 10% of 450?

Step 1. What is 10% of 450?
↑ ↑ ↑
Part | Whole
Percent

Step 2. Percent → $\dfrac{10}{100} = \dfrac{x}{450}$ ← Part
← Whole

Step 3. $\dfrac{10}{100} = \dfrac{x}{450}$

$$100x = (10)(450)$$

$$\dfrac{100x}{100} = \dfrac{(10)(450)}{100}$$

$$x = 45$$

Step 4. Check. $\dfrac{10}{100} = \dfrac{45}{450}$

$$(10)(450) = (45)(100)$$

$$4500 = 4500$$

(b) 17 is what % of 68?

Step 1. 17 is what % of 68
↑ ↑ ↑
Part | Whole
Percent

Step 2. Percent → $\dfrac{x}{100} = \dfrac{17}{68}$ ← Part
← Whole

Step 3. $\dfrac{x}{100} = \dfrac{17}{68}$

$$68x = (17)(100)$$

$$\dfrac{68x}{68} = \dfrac{(17)(100)}{68}$$

$$x = 25$$

$$\dfrac{25}{100} = 25\%$$

3.4. The Percent Proportion

Step 4. Check. $\dfrac{25}{100} = \dfrac{17}{68}$

$(25)(68) = (17)(100)$

$1700 = 1700$

(c) Cimetidine is a drug that can produce side effects such as dizziness and a rash. The number of people who experience these side effects is about 1% of all those who take the drug. If 1500 people take cimetidine, how many persons are expected to experience the side effects?

Step 1. Translate the words into a percent statement.

What is 1% of 1500?

Step 2. Set up the percent proportion and solve.

Percent → $\dfrac{1}{100} = \dfrac{x}{1500}$ ← Part
← Whole

Step 3. $100x = (1)(1500)$

$\dfrac{100x}{100} = \dfrac{(1)(1500)}{100}$

$x = 15$ Fifteen people will probably suffer the side effects of cimetidine.

Step 4. Check. $\dfrac{1}{100} = \dfrac{15}{1500}$

$(1)(1500) = (15)(100)$

$1500 = 1500$

(d) A 25-kg child is to receive a dose of isotonic sodium chloride equivalent to 2% of her body weight. Calculate in kg the correct amount of isotonic sodium chloride to be administered to this patient.

Step 1. Translate the words into a percent statement.

What is 2% of 25 kg?

Step 2. Set up the percent proportion and solve.

Percent → $\dfrac{2}{100} = \dfrac{x}{25}$ ← Part
← Whole

Step 3.
$$100x = (2)(25)$$
$$\frac{100x}{100} = \frac{(2)(25)}{100}$$
$$x = \frac{1}{2}$$

Answer. Administer $\frac{1}{2}$ kg of isotonic sodium chloride to the child.

Step 4. Check.
$$\frac{2}{100} = \frac{\frac{1}{2}}{25}$$
$$\left(\frac{1}{2}\right)(100) = (2)(25)$$
$$50 = 50$$

PRACTICE SET 3.4

Identify the percent, whole, and part in each of the following percent questions.

1. 10 is what % of 500?

2. 35% of what number is 42?

3. What number is 0.6% of 44?

Solve each of the following percent problems. Round off the answers to the nearest tenth.

4. 6% of what number is 70?

5. What % of 300 is 60?

6. A 20-kg child has been prescribed isotonic sodium chloride equivalent to $2\frac{1}{2}$% of her body weight. How many kg of isotonic sodium chloride should be administered to the child?

7. A 5% solution of hydrogen peroxide has been prepared by the pharmacist. If the total amount prepared is 10 milliliters (mL), how many mL are pure drug.

8. 100 oz of a 0.5% glycerol solution are on hand in the stock room. How many oz of this solution are pure glycerol?

9. 5 liters (L) of 10% Burow's solution have been prepared for use in the hospital. How many L of concentrated Burow's solution does this 10% solution contain?

10. Some side effects of Tagamet, a drug used to treat duodenal ulcers, are dizziness, diarrhea, muscular pain, and a rash. Tests have indicated that approximately 1% of all patients treated with Tagamet experience these side effects. If 500 people were treated with Tagamet, how many people experienced these side effects?

3.5 CHAPTER 3 REVIEW PROBLEMS

Write each of the following comparisons in both colon and fractional forms.

1. 8 to 5 **2.** 7.3 to 1 **3.** $2\frac{1}{2}$ to 100

4. 100 mg testosterone propionate per mL

5. 6 g/m^2

Indicate if each proportion is true or false.

6. $\dfrac{3}{8} \stackrel{?}{=} \dfrac{6}{16}$ **7.** $\dfrac{12}{1\frac{3}{4}} \stackrel{?}{=} \dfrac{48}{7}$ **8.** $\dfrac{9}{8.5} \stackrel{?}{=} \dfrac{7}{6}$

Solve and check each proportion. Round off each decimal answer to the nearest tenth.

9. $\dfrac{5}{9} = \dfrac{x}{117}$ **10.** $\dfrac{x}{98} = \dfrac{5}{7}$

11. $\dfrac{x}{3} = \dfrac{2\frac{1}{2}}{8}$ **12.** $\dfrac{9}{26} = \dfrac{x}{4\frac{1}{3}}$

13. $\dfrac{x}{100} = \dfrac{74}{200}$ **14.** $\dfrac{x}{7} = \dfrac{9}{0.6}$

15. $\dfrac{x}{1} = \dfrac{0.5}{1.5}$

Solve each of the following word problems using proportions.

16. A physician orders 45 mL of Milk of Magnesia for a patient. If there are 30 mL in 1 oz, how many oz should be given to the patient?

17. A preoperative order calls for 0.5 mg of atropine sulfate. The bottle is labeled 0.4 mg per cc. How many cc should be given?

18. A physician orders digoxin elixir, 0.035 mg, for a child. If the label on the bottle reads 0.05 mg/mL, how many mL should be given?

19. Calcium lactate, 15 g/m^2 body surface, is prescribed for a patient. How many g should be given to a patient with a body surface of 1.45 m^2?

20. A child weighs 22 kg. If a doctor prescribes 0.35 mg of medicine per kg body mass, how many mg should be administered?

Convert each of the following percent forms to its equivalent decimal form.

21. 14%

22. 6%

23. 0.7%

24. 0.02%

25. 15.8%

Convert each of the following decimals to its equivalent percent.

26. 0.47

27. 0.03

28. 3.5

29. 7.28

30. 0.0082

Solve each of the following percent problems. Round off each decimal to the nearest tenth.

31. 60% of what number is 78?

32. 11 is what % of 33?

33. What number is 42% of 150?

34. 7.9 is what % of 39.5?

35. $87\frac{1}{2}$% of what number is 49?

36. Lomotil is a drug used to treat patients suffering from diarrhea. In a certain study, 5% of 300 people showed no positive results while being treated with a Lomotil. How many people did not show positive results?

37. A certain study reveals that 3% of all patients suffer side effects from a certain drug. If 5500 people take the drug, how many are expected to experience the side effects?

38. 15% of a certain sodium chloride solution is considered to be pure sodium chloride. How many parts are considered to be pure sodium chloride in a 500 mL solution?

39. A 10 mL 1% solution of gentian violet has been prescribed by a doctor to be rubbed on a patient's affected area between the toes three times daily. How many parts of this 1% gentian violet solution are pure gentian violet?

40. 50 mL of 0.5% hydrocortisone in lotion has been prescribed for a patient and is applied to her rash twice daily. How many parts of this hydrocortisone solution are pure hydrocortisone?

3.6 CHAPTER 3 SELF TEST

3.1 Write the following comparison in both colon and fractional forms.

1. $3\frac{1}{2}$ to 100 _____ _____

3.2 Solve each proportion.

2. $\dfrac{1}{65} = \dfrac{2}{x}$ _____

3. $\dfrac{x}{1} = \dfrac{0.5}{15}$ _____

4. $\dfrac{8}{100} = \dfrac{x}{\frac{1}{4}}$ _____

3.2 Solve each of the following word problems using proportions. Round off the answers to the nearest tenth.

5. A doctor's order reads, "Administer 50 mg amobarbital." Amobarbital is available as an elixir, 22 mg per 5 mL. How many mL will you administer? _____

6. A preoperative order calls for atropine sulfate, 0.55 mg. If the bottle is labeled 0.25 mg/cc, how many cc will you administer? _____

7. The doctor prescribes 15 mg digoxin per kg body mass for a 24-kg child. How many mg should be administered? _____

3.3 Convert the following percent to its equivalent decimal form.

8. 0.5% _____

3.3 Convert each of the following numbers to its equivalent percent.

9. 0.93 _____

10. 0.003 _____

3.4 Solve each of the following percent problems. Round answer to the nearest tenth.

11. What number is 16% of 38? _____

12. 8.2% of what number is 12.3? _____

13. 25% of a certain solution is considered to be pure drug. How many mL of an 800 mL solution would be pure drug? _____

14. 10% of all patients who take a certain drug experience side effects. If 500 people take this particular drug, how many people are expected to experience side effects? _____

15. 350 mL of a 1.5% neomycin irrigation solution are ordered. How many parts of the 350 mL would be the neomycin drug? _____

SUMMARY OF CHAPTER 3 RULES

RULE 3.1 Cross Products Rule
If two fractions are equivalent, their cross products are equal.

RULE 3.2 Cross Product Equality Rule
If the cross products of two fractions in a proportion are equal, then the fractions are equivalent. The proportion is true.

Summary of Chapter 3 Rules

RULE 3.3 Rule of Equality for Addition

If the same number is added to each member of an equality, the sums are equal.

If $a = b$, then $a + c = b + c$

RULE 3.4 Rule of Equality for Subtraction

If the same number is subtracted from each member of an equality, the differences are equal.

If $a = b$, then $a - c = b - c$

RULE 3.5 Rule of Equality for Multiplication

If each member of an equality is multiplied by the same number, the products are equal.

If $a = b$, then $ac = bc$

RULE 3.6 Rule of Equality for Division

If each member of an equality is divided by the same number (zero excluded), the quotients are equal.

If $a = b$ and $c \neq 0$, then $\dfrac{a}{c} = \dfrac{b}{c}$.

RULE 3.7 Rule for Solving a Proportion

Step 1. Write the cross products in equation form.

Step 2. Divide each member by the number that multiplies the unknown letter. (Use the rule of equality for division.)

Step 3. Simplify the equation.

RULE 3.8 Medication Rule

Ratio for Medication on Hand = Ratio for Desired Medication
    (MOH)   (DM)

RULE 3.9 Rule for Converting a Percent to Its Equivalent Decimal Form

To change from a percent form to a decimal form, multiply by 0.01; that is, move the decimal point two places to the left.

RULE 3.10 Rule for Solving a Percent Proportion

Step 1. Identify the three categories of the percent statement: the percent, the whole, and the part.

Step 2. Set the percent, whole, and part into the percent proportion:
$$\frac{\text{percent}}{100} = \frac{\text{part}}{\text{whole}}$$
Represent the unknown quantity by x.

Step 3. Solve the proportion for the unknown quantity x.

Step 4. Check the solution.

PART II Clinical Calculations

4
The Metric System of Measurement

OBJECTIVES

After studying this chapter, you should be able to

1. read and write units in the metric system;
2. convert from one metric unit to another;
3. convert between Celsius and Fahrenheit scales;
4. solve practical problems involving metric units.

INTRODUCTION

The metric system was developed by the French in the latter part of the eighteenth century and was officially adopted in France in 1799. The system, based on the decimal scale, was made to be precise and simple.

Although Congress declared in 1866 that the metric system was the official measurement system of the United States, the use of the metric system was not made mandatory. Therefore, it has been used only partially in the United States, having been adopted particularly in the sciences and pharmacies, in weighing currency at the federal mints, and in the armed forces.

The updated metric system (1961) is based on the wavelength of light of krypton-86 and on the mass of a cylinder of platinum-iridium alloy. This modern metric system provides more accurate definitions of the basic metric units. This system is called the International System of Units (abbreviated SI for the French name, Système, International d'Unites). About 92% of the countries of the world use this SI system.

Because the field of medical science has adopted the SI, it is imperative that you understand it and feel confident in using it.

4.1 THE BASIC METRIC UNITS OF MEASURE

The three basic metric units used in the medical field are:

meter, denoting length (m)

liter, denoting volume (L)

gram, denoting mass (g)

Other units are formed by adding Latin or Greek prefixes to the names of these basic units. Latin prefixes are used to designate fractional parts of the basic unit: deci- (0.1), centi- (0.01), milli- (0.001), and micro- (0.000001). Greek prefixes are used to designate the multiples of the basic units: deka- (10), hecto- (100), and kilo- (1000). The most commonly used metric units are the kilo-, centi-, milli- and micro-.

Table 4-1 on page 81 provides the complete table of metric prefixes.

The prefixes, their abbreviations, and their positions in the table should be memorized. In the vertical columns in Table 4-1, each unit has a value 10 times the value of the unit immediately below it. In other words, it takes 10 of any unit to make one of the unit directly above it. For example:

10 milli- = 1 centi-

10 centi- = 1 deci-

10 deci- = 1 m, L, g

10 m, L, g = 1 deka-

10 deka- = 1 hecto-

10 hecto- = 1 kilo-

There are two units of 10 between milli- and micro-. Although they are unnamed here, when converting from one metric unit to another be sure to consider these unnamed levels. They do affect the position of the decimal point.

The basic unit of length is the **meter** (m). It is approximately 39.4 in., or about 3 in. longer than a yardstick. Figure 4-1 shows the metric ruler. Table 4-2 shows the metric length relationships.

4.1. The Basic Metric Units of Measure

TABLE 4-1 METRIC PREFIXES

Prefix	Abbreviation	Denotes
kilo-	k	1000 units
hecto-	h	100 units
deka-	da	10 units
	L, g, m	1 basic unit
deci-	d	0.1 unit
centi-	c	0.01 unit
milli-	m	0.001 unit
micro-	mc (μ)	0.000001 unit

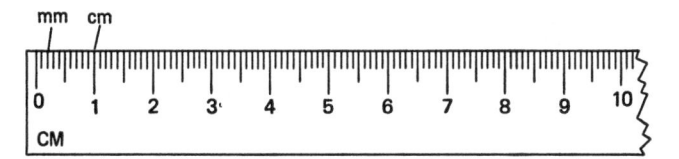

Figure 4-1 Metric ruler

TABLE 4-2 TABLE OF METRIC LENGTHS

Unit	Abbreviation	Denotes
kilometer	km	1000 m
hectometer	hm	100 m
dekameter	dam	10 m
meter	m	1 m
decimeter	dm	0.1 m
centimeter	cm	0.01 m
millimeter	mm	0.001 m
micrometer	mcm (μm)	0.000001 m

The **liter** (L), in health-related occupations, is the basic unit of volume. Even though it is not an official SI unit, it is defined in terms of metric and is accepted as the basic unit of volume. Since it is approximately equal to a quart (1.06 qt), for practical purposes it can be said that 1 L equals 1 qt. Table 4-3 shows the metric volume relationships. Figure 4-2 shows the liter-quart relationship.

TABLE 4–3 TABLE OF METRIC VOLUMES

Unit	Abbreviation	Denotes
kiloliter	kL	1000 L
hectoliter	hL	100 L
dekaliter	daL	10 L
liter	L	1 L
deciliter	dL	0.1 L
centiliter	cL	0.01 L
milliliter	mL	0.001 L
microliter	mcL (μL)	0.000001 L

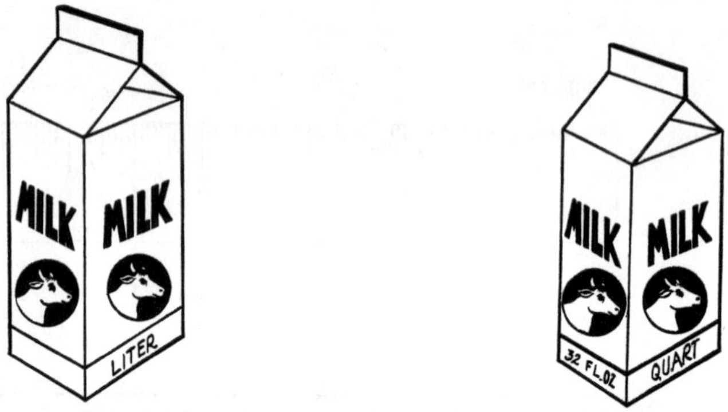

1 Liter 1 Quart

Figure 4–2 A liter comparison

The medical field accepts the **gram** (g) as the basic unit of mass, even though the official SI unit is the kilogram. Table 4–4 shows the metric mass relationships. Figure 4–3 shows some gram comparisons.

TABLE 4–4 TABLE OF METRIC MASSES

Unit	Abbreviation	Denotes
kilogram	kg	1000 g
hectogram	hg	100 g
dekagram	dag	10 g
gram	g	1 g
decigram	dg	0.1 g
centigram	cg	0.01 g
milligram	mg	0.001 g
microgram	mcg (μg)	0.000001 g

4.1. The Basic Metric Units of Measure

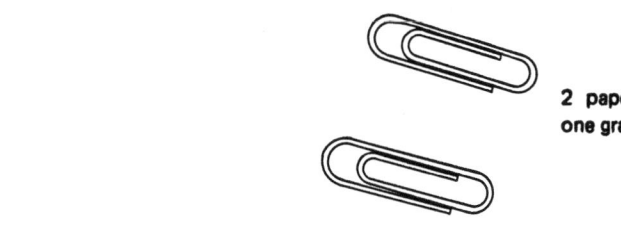

2 paper clips weigh approximately one gram.

A pencil weighs about five grams.

Figure 4–3 Gram comparisons

EXAMPLE 4.1

Write another metric abbreviation for 10 g.
Since the prefix for 10 is deka-, 10 g equals 1 dag.

Answer. 10 g = 1 dag

EXAMPLE 4.2

Write another metric abbreviation for 1000 L.
Since the prefix for 1000 is kilo-, 1000 L equals 1 kL.

Answer. 1000 L = 1 kL

EXAMPLE 4.3

Write another metric abbreviation for 0.1 m.
Since the prefix for 0.1 is deci-, 0.1 m equals 1 dm.

Answer. 0.1 m = 1 dm

EXAMPLE 4.4

0.001 m = 1 _____ ?
The prefix for 0.001 is milli-.

Answer. 0.001 m = 1 mm

EXAMPLE 4.5

Write 1 cm using the *basic unit* of length.
Centi- means 0.01 of a unit. Therefore 1 cm equals .01 m.

Answer. 1 cm = 0.01 m

PRACTICE SET 4.1

Write the correct abbreviations for problems 1–5.

1. 1000 grams = _____
2. 0.000001 liter = _____
3. 0.01 meter = _____
4. 0.001 meter = _____
5. 10 grams = _____
6. A decigram = _____ g
7. A microliter = _____ L
8. A millimeter = _____ m
9. A kilometer = _____ m
10. A dekagram = _____ g
11. It takes _____ cg to make a gram.
12. It takes _____ mL to make a liter.

4.2 METRIC CONVERSIONS

It has been stated that the metric system is a decimal system. Therefore, the same power-of-10 relationship exists in the metric system as exists in the decimal numeration system. To change from one unit to another means multiplying or dividing by a power of 10. Multiplication and division by powers of 10 can be performed by relocating the decimal point. For example, to divide a number by 10, the decimal point in the original number can be moved one place value to the left.

EXAMPLE 4.6

$$83.0 \div 10 = 8.3.0$$

↑
Original
decimal
point

Relocation of decimal point
one place value to the left

To divide a number by 1000, the decimal point can be relocated three place values to the left of the place it occupied in the original number.

4.2. Metric Conversions

EXAMPLE 4.7

$$459.1 \div 1000 = 0.459.1$$

↑
Original decimal point

Decimal point relocated three places to the left

The decimal point is relocated as many places to the left of the original place in the dividend as there are zeros in the divisor. In Example 4.6, the decimal point was relocated one place to the left in the dividend, since there was one zero in the divisor (10). In Example 4.7, the decimal point was relocated three places to the left in the dividend, since there were three zeros in the divisor (1000).

EXAMPLE 4.8

$1547 \div 100 =$

$1547. \div 100 =$

↑   ↑
Original   Two zeros   Relocate decimal two places to the left
decimal
point

$1547 \div 100 = 15.47.$

Relocated decimal

Answer. $1547 \div 100 = 15.47$

In multiplication, the decimal point is relocated to the right of the original decimal point rather than to the left. To multiply by a power of 10, the decimal point in the product is relocated to the right as many decimal places as there are zeros in the multiplier.

EXAMPLE 4.9

$45.91 \times 10 =$

$45.91 \times 10 =$

↑   ↑
Original   One zero   Relocate decimal one place value to the right in the product.
decimal
point

$45.91 \times 10 = 49.9.1$

Relocated decimal point

Answer. $45.91 \times 10 = 459.1$

EXAMPLE 4.10

$15 \times 1000 =$

$\underset{\underset{\text{Original decimal point}}{\uparrow}}{15.} \times \underset{\underset{\text{Three zeros}}{\uparrow}}{1000} =$ Relocate decimal three places to the right in the product.

$15. \times 1000 = 15.000.$

Add zeros so that decimal point can be relocated three places.

Answer. $15 \times 1000 = 15{,}000$

These rules can be applied to the metric system, since in each vertical column each unit has a value 10 times the value of the unit immediately below it. Changing from one metric unit to another in the same table can be accomplished by relocating the decimal point; that is, mulitplying or dividing by 10 or powers of 10. Arrange the metric prefixes on a horizontal line so that the decimal point can be moved to the left or right, just as was done with the decimal numerals.

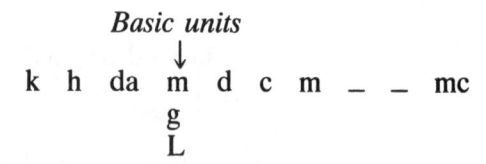

Basic units
↓
k   h   da   m   d   c   m   _   _   mc
           g
           L

Depending on whether you multiply or divide by a power of 10, changing from one metric unit to another requires relocating the decimal point to the right or to the left. You may become confused as to whether to multiply or divide when changing from one metric unit to another; therefore, the following rule has been devised so that you will make no mistake converting from one unit to another.

RULE 4.1 Rule for Metric Conversion

Step 1. Write the horizontal metric scale.

Step 2. Circle the two units stated in the problem.

Step 3. Count the number of metric units from the unit given to the unit desired. Note the direction.

Step 4. Move the decimal point the number of places counted in Step 3 and in the direction noted.

4.2. Metric Conversions	87

EXAMPLE 4.11

Change 1 000.0 mm to m.

Step 1. Write the horizontal metric scale.

$$k \quad h \quad da \quad \begin{matrix}g\\m\\L\end{matrix} \quad d \quad c \quad m \quad \_ \quad \_ \quad mc$$

Step 2. Circle the two units stated in the problem.

$$k \quad h \quad da \quad \begin{matrix}g\\ \textcircled{m}\\L\end{matrix} \quad d \quad c \quad \textcircled{m} \quad \_ \quad \_ \quad mc$$

Step 3. Meter is three units to the left of milli.

$$k \quad h \quad da \quad \begin{matrix}g\\ \textcircled{m}\\L\end{matrix} \quad d \quad c \quad \textcircled{m} \quad \_ \quad \_ \quad mc$$

Step 4. Move the decimal point in 1000.0 three places to the left.

$$1\,.\,000\,.\,0$$

Answer. 1 000.0 mm = 1 m

EXAMPLE 4.12

Change 6.9 kL to dL.

Steps 1. and 2.

$$\textcircled{k} \quad h \quad da \quad \begin{matrix}g\\m\\L\end{matrix} \quad \textcircled{d} \quad c \quad m \quad \_ \quad \_ \quad mc$$

Step 3.

$$\textcircled{k} \quad h \quad da \quad \begin{matrix}g\\m\\L\end{matrix} \quad \textcircled{d} \quad c \quad m \quad \_ \quad \_ \quad mc$$

d is four places to the right of k

Step 4. Move the decimal point four places to the right.

$$6\,.\,9000\,.$$

Answer. 6.9 kL = 69 000 dL

EXAMPLE 4.13

Change 10 g to mcg.

Steps 1, 2, 3.

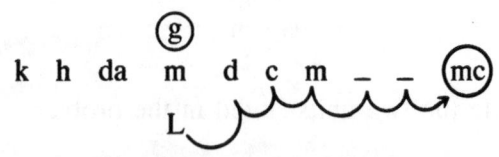

k h da m d c m _ _ mc
        (g)
        L

Six places to the right

Step 4. Move the decimal point six places to the right.

10.000000.   (add zeros as needed)

Answer. 10 g = 10 000 000 mcg

PRACTICE SET 4.2

1. Change 50 g to mg. _____
2. Change 3 mm to m. _____
3. Change 0.002 kL to L. _____
4. Change 1.2 g to kg. _____
5. Change 140 m to mcm. _____
6. 0.6 mg = _____ mcg
7. 346 hg = _____ dag
8. 14.16 cm = _____ m
9. 1678 mcm = _____ m
10. 0.05 kg = _____ g

There are interrelationships among length, mass, and volume in the metric system. The study of these interrelationships begins with the cubic centimeter. A cubic centimeter (cm^3) is a cube whose length, width, and height are 1 cm. (See Fig. 4–4.) The formula for the volume of a cube is

$$V = (length)(width)(height).$$

The volume for this cube is

$$V = (1 \text{ cm})(1 \text{ cm})(1 \text{ cm}) = 1 \text{ cm}^3.$$

4.3. Temperature Scales

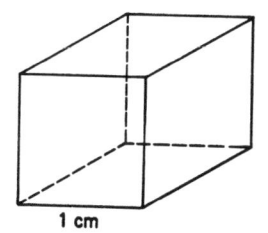

Figure 4-4 A cubic centimeter

The cm³ is often referred to as a **cc**, and the terms are used interchangeably. At sea level and at 4°C, 1 cc contains 1 mL of distilled water and weighs approximately 1 g. Therefore, it can be said that under these standard conditions, the following relationship exists:

$$1 \text{ cc} \approx 1 \text{ mL} \approx 1 \text{ g}$$

In health-related occupations, this relationship is used not only for water but also for water-based solutions.

4.3 TEMPERATURE SCALES

Both the Celsius (°C) and the Fahrenheit (°F) scales are used to measure temperature. On the Fahrenheit scale, the boiling point of water is 212°, and the freezing point of water is 32°. This is an interval of 180° (212° − 32°). On the Celsius scale, the interval between the boiling point of water (100°) and the freezing point (0°) is 100° (100° − 0°). Figure 4-5 compares the two scales.

In some hospitals today, a patient's body temperature is measured using the Fahrenheit scale, although the trend is toward using the Celsius scale. You should be familiar with both temperature scales and be able to convert between the two scales, if necessary.

The ratio of the boiling-freezing interval for the two scales is

$$\text{Celsius: } 100° - 0° = 100° \longrightarrow \frac{100°}{180°} = \frac{5}{9}$$
$$\text{Fahrenheit: } 212° - 32° = 180°$$

The rule for converting between the °F and the °C scales is based on this ratio of $\frac{5}{9}$.

RULE 4.2 Conversion for the °F−°C Scales

$$\frac{°C}{°F - 32°} = \frac{5}{9}$$

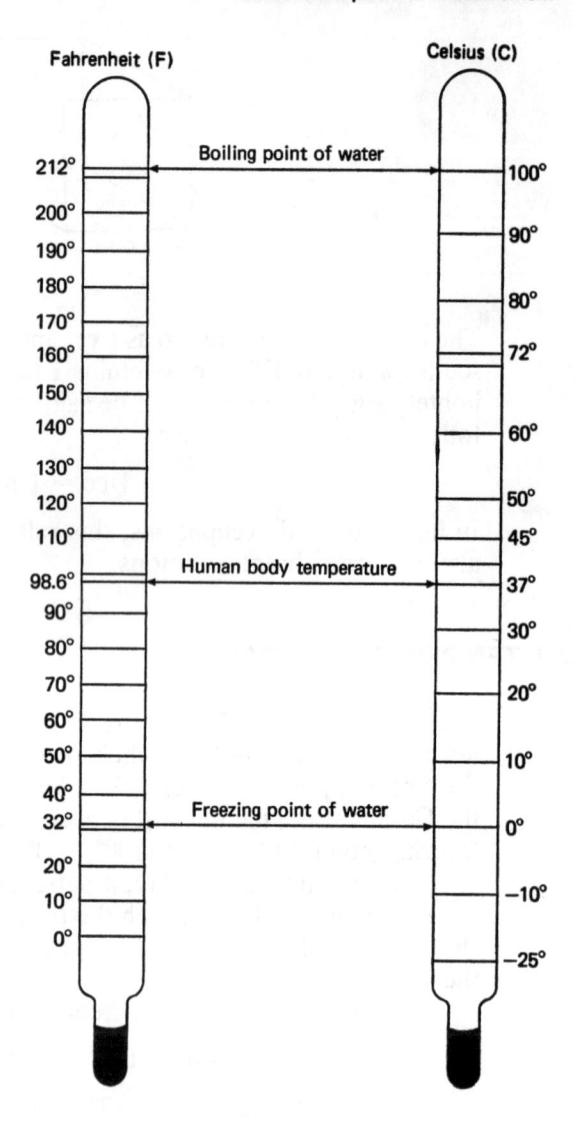

Figure 4-5 Comparison of the Fahrenheit and Celsius scales

EXAMPLE 4.14

Convert 140°F to °C.

Use Rule 4.2.

$$\frac{°C}{°F - 32°} = \frac{5}{9}$$

4.3. Temperature Scales

Substitute 140° for °F.

$$\frac{°C}{140° - 32°} = \frac{5}{9}$$

Solve the proportion.

$$(9)(°C) = (140° - 32°)(5)$$
$$9(°C) = (108°)(5)$$
$$9(°C) = 540°$$
$$\frac{(9)(°C)}{9} = \frac{540°}{9}$$

Answer. $\quad °C = 60°$

EXAMPLE 4.15

Convert 200°C to °F.

Substitute in the conversion equation.

$$°C \rightarrow \frac{200°}{°F - 32°} = \frac{5}{9}$$

When obtaining the cross products, the 5 multiplies both the °F and the 32. $(5)(°F - 32°) = 5°F - 160°$. This is called the distributive property for multiplication.

Solve the proportion.

$$5(°F - 32°) = (9)(200°)$$
$$5°F - 160° = 1800° \qquad \text{Cross products.}$$
$$5°F - 160° + 160° = 1800° + 160° \qquad \text{Add 160° to both sides.}$$
$$5°F + 0 = 1960° \qquad \text{Simplify.}$$
$$5°F = 1960°$$
$$\frac{5°F}{5} = \frac{1960°}{5} \qquad \text{Divide both sides by 5.}$$

Answer. $\quad °F = 392°$

EXAMPLE 4.16

Convert 120°C to °F.

Substitute in the conversion equation.

$$°C \rightarrow \frac{120°}{°F - 32°} = \frac{5}{9}$$

$$5(°F - 32°) = (9)(120°)$$
$$5°F - 160° = 1080°$$
$$5°F - 160° + 160° = 1080° + 160°$$
$$5°F = 1240°$$
$$\frac{5°F}{5} = \frac{1240°}{5}$$

Answer. $°F = 248°$

PRACTICE SET 4.3

1. Convert 60°C to °F.
2. Convert 482°F to °C.
3. Convert 50°F to °C.
4. Convert 43.5°C to °F.
5. Convert 125.6°F to °C.

4.4 METRIC UNITS AND THEIR APPLICATIONS

Once the metric system has been mastered, it is important that you be able to apply it to practical situations.

A basic medication rule (Rule 4.3) can be used for many medication problems. This is the same rule as Rule 3.8.

RULE 4.3   Medication Rule

Ratio for medication on hand = Ratio for desired medication

(MOH = DM)

4.4. Metric Units and Their Applications

The medication on hand (MOH) is defined as the drug available in the supply room or from the pharmacist. The desired medication (DM) is the amount of drug prescribed by the physician to be administered to the patient.

EXAMPLE 4.17

Desired medication: 4000 mg magnesium carbonate.
Medication on hand: 2 g tabs magnesium carbonate. How many magnesium carbonate tablets will you administer?

Use Rule 4.3:

$$\underset{\downarrow}{\text{Medication on hand}} = \underset{\downarrow}{\text{Desired medication}}$$

$$\frac{2 \text{ g}}{1 \text{ tab}} = \frac{4000 \text{ mg}}{x \text{ tabs}}$$

Before this proportion can be solved, like units must appear in the numerators of the two ratios, and like units must appear in the denominators. A good rule of thumb to follow is to change the unit label of the desired medication so that it agrees with the unit label of the medication on hand. Change the 4000 mg to g.

$$4000 \text{ mg} = 4 \text{ g}$$

Then substitute the converted quantity into the proportion.

$$\underset{\downarrow}{\text{MOH}} = \underset{\downarrow}{\text{DM}}$$

$$\frac{2 \text{ g}}{1 \text{ tab}} = \frac{4 \text{ g}}{x \text{ tabs}} \leftarrow 4000 \text{ mg}$$

$$2x = 4$$

Answer. $x = 2$ tabs magnesium carbonate (2g/tab)

EXAMPLE 4.18

Desired medication: 450 mcg. Medication on hand: .3 mg scored tabs. How many tabs will you administer?

Use Rule 4.3:

$$\underset{\downarrow}{\text{MOH}} = \underset{\downarrow}{\text{DM}}$$

$$\frac{0.3 \text{ mg}}{1 \text{ tab}} = \frac{450 \text{ mcg}}{x \text{ tabs}}$$

Before this proportion can be solved, like units must appear in the numerators.

Since they do not have like units, change the desired medication, 450 mcg, to the units of the medication on hand, mg.

$$450 \text{ mcg} = .450 \text{ mg}$$

Substitute the converted quantity into the proportion.

$$\underset{\downarrow}{\text{MOH}} = \underset{\downarrow}{\text{DM}}$$

$$\frac{0.3 \text{ mg}}{1 \text{ tab}} = \frac{0.45 \text{ mg}}{x \text{ tabs}} \leftarrow 450 \text{ mcg}$$

$$0.3x = 0.45$$

Answer. $x = 1.5$ tabs of the 0.3 mg/tab drug.

EXAMPLE 4.19

A doctor prescribes .3 g simethicone total daily to be administred in four equally divided doses. Simethicone comes in 20 mg, 25 mg, 40 mg, and 60 mg tabs. How many tabs, of which strength, should you administer per dose?

Divide the problem into three parts.

Part 1. Change the 0.3 g desired medication to mg, since all the available tablets come in mg units.

$$0.3 \text{ g} = 300 \text{ mg}$$

Part 2. Since the medication is to be administered in four equally divided doses, find the amount of one dose.

$$300 \text{ mg} \div 4 \text{ doses} = 75 \text{ mg/dose}$$

Part 3. Compare the strengths of the available tabs. Three 25 mg tabs per dose would satisfy the doctor's order.

Answer. Administer three 25 mg tabs of simethicone per dose.

It is best to give a patient the least number of tabs. Therefore, the strongest strengths, when possible, should be used. Tablets should not be divided unless they are scored.

EXAMPLE 4.20

A doctor prescribes 2 g/m^2 body surface of a syrup for a patient who has a body surface of 0.9 m^2. The syrup is available as 500 mg/5 mL. How many mL should you administer?

Divide the problem into two parts.

Part 1. Find the number of grams needed for the patient, based on the patient's body surface.

$$\underset{\text{by doctor}}{\text{Amount prescribed}} = \underset{\text{by patient}}{\text{Amount needed}}$$

$$\frac{2 \text{ g}}{1 \text{ m}^2} = \frac{x \text{ g}}{0.9 \text{ m}^2}$$

$$x = 1.8 \text{ g}$$

Part 2. Find the number of mL to be administered to the patient.

$$\underset{\downarrow}{\text{MOH}} = \underset{\downarrow}{\text{DM}}$$

$$\frac{500 \text{ mg}}{5 \text{ mL}} = \frac{1.8 \text{ g}}{x \text{ mL}}$$

By substitution:

$$\underset{\downarrow}{\text{MOH}} = \underset{\downarrow}{\text{DM}}$$

$$\frac{500 \text{ mg}}{5 \text{ mL}} = \frac{1800 \text{ mg}}{x \text{ mL}} \leftarrow \text{1.8 g changed to mg}$$

$$500x = (5)(1800)$$
$$500x = 9000$$
$$x = 18 \text{ mL}$$

Answer. Administer 18 mL of the syrup (500 mg/5 mL).

PRACTICE SET 4.4

1. A doctor orders erythromycin 1000 mg daily in four equally divided doses. Erythromycin comes in 0.25 g/tab, 1 g/tab, and 2.5 g/tab. How many tabs, of which strength, will you give per dose?

2. Desired medication: 0.04 mg. Medication on hand: 30 mcg/cc. How many cc will you administer?

3. A doctor orders Flagyl 50 mg/kg body mass for a patient. The patient weighs 54 kg. How many g will the patient receive?

4. A doctor prescribes indocyanine green 1.5 mg/kg body mass. If indocyanine green is available as 0.01 g/cc, how many cc would you give to a 70-kg patient?

5. Ordered: Sodium bicarbonate 0.9 g. On hand: Sodium bicarbonate tabs of 300 mg and 600 mg. Which strength(s) and how many tabs will you administer?

4.5 CHAPTER 4 REVIEW PROBLEMS

Convert the following to the indicated units.

1. 302°F = _____ °C
2. 3.25 L = _____ mL
3. 0.001 mL = _____ mcL
4. 85 432 mL = _____ daL
5. 0.00795 kg = _____ g
6. 35 000 mcg = _____ g
7. 5.5 L = _____ cm^3
8. 60°C = _____ °F
9. 250 cc = _____ mL
10. 1.9 mL = _____ L
11. 130°F = _____ °C
12. 4.5 mL = _____ g
13. 5 km = _____ mm
14. 73.2°C = _____ °F
15. 395 cm^3 = _____ L
16. 59 L = _____ cc
17. 14.5 mcL = _____ L
18. 86°F = _____ °C
19. 250°C = _____ °F
20. 2000 mcL = _____ mL
21. 1.6 L = _____ kL
22. 0.008 m = _____ cm

4.5. Chapter 4 Review Problems

23. 9540 g = _____ kg

24. 1000 cc = _____ mL

25. 1000 cm³ = _____ L

26. Deltasone 0.08 g total is to be given daily in four equally divided doses. Deltasone tabs come in 2.5 mg, 5 mg, 10 mg, and 50 mg tabs. How many tabs of which kind will you give per dose?

27. Gantrisin syrup 2 g/m² body surface has been ordered for a patient with a body surface of 0.75 m². If Gantrisin 500 mg/5 cc is available, how many cc will you administer?

28. Desired medication: 400 mg magnesium carbonate. Medication on hand: 0.2 g tabs magnesium carbonate. How many tabs will you administer?

29. Administer hydrocodone bitartrate 0.02 g/m² body surface, daily in three divided doses. The body surface of the patient is 0.8 m². Hydrocodone bitartrate comes in 5 mg/5 cc strength. How many cc will you administer per dose?

30. Sodium bicarbonate 1.2 g is needed. Sodium bicarbonate tabs in 300 mg, 500 mg, and 600 mg doses are available. Which strength tabs will you use, and how many will you administer?

31. 3.6 g aspirin has been ordered daily in four divided doses. Aspirin tabs come in 300 mg, 325 mg, 400 mg, and 450 mg tab strengths. How many tabs and of which strength will you administer per dose?

32. Order: 0.03 mg. Medication on hand: 15 mcg/cc. How many cc will you administer?

33. Order: 300 mcg. Medication on hand: 0.2 mg scored tabs. How many tabs will you administer?

34. Desired medication: 6 g methionine total daily in four divided doses. Medication on hand: 500 mg tabs methionine. How many methionine tabs will you give per dose?

35. Desired medication: Methyclothiazide 150 mcg/kg of body mass. How many tabs will you administer to a 50-kg patient if methyclothiazide tabs come in 2.5 mg, 3.5 mg, and 4 mg scored tabs? Which strengths?

36. Desired medication: 150 mcg; Medication on hand: 0.03 mg/tab. How many tabs will you administer?

37. Desired medication: 0.4 g methionine total daily in two equally divided doses. Medication on hand: 200 mg tablets. How many methionine tabs will you administer per dose?

38. Methyclothiazide 100 mcg/kg body mass has been ordered for a 35-kg patient. Methyclothiazide tablets 3.5 mg scored and 5 mg scored are available. Which one(s) will you administer?

39. Gantrisin syrup 3 g/m² body surface has been ordered for a patient with a 0.6 m² body surface. If Gantrisin syrup 0.5 g/5 cc is available, how many cc will you administer?

40. Order: Diphemanil methylsulfate 1.5 g daily in three equally divided doses. Medication on hand: diphemanil methylsulfate 250 mg tabs. How many tabs will you administer per dose?

4.6 CHAPTER 4 SELF TEST

Fill in the blanks:

4.2	**1.** 0.005 kg =	_____ g
4.2	**2.** 412 mL =	_____ cc
4.3	**3.** 50°F =	_____ °C
4.2	**4.** 3500 mL =	_____ L
4.2	**5.** 100°C =	_____ °F
4.2	**6.** 5 L =	_____ cc
4.3	**7.** 30°C =	_____ °F
4.2	**8.** 250 mcL =	_____ g
4.2	**9.** 0.15 hm =	_____ dm
4.2	**10.** 0.00075 m =	_____ mcm

Solve for the information requested. Be sure to label your answers.

4.4 **11.** Desired medication: 600 mg. Medication on hand: 0.5 g/cc. How many cc will you administer?

4.4 **12.** A doctor prescribes Benadryl 0.05 g 3 times a day for two days. Benadryl is available from the pharmacy in 25 mg capsules. How many capsules should you order for two days?

4.4 **13.** A patient is to receive Valium 30 mg daily in three equally divided doses. The available tabs are 5 mg/tab, 2 mg/tab, and 1 mg/tab. Which strength and how many should you administer per dose?

4.4 **14.** Methyclothiazide scored tabs are available in 2.5 mg/tab and 5 mg/tab. A doctor prescribes 100 mcg/kg body mass for a patient weighing 50 kg. Which strength and how many should you administer? _____

4.4 **15.** A physician orders Achromycin for a patient who has a surface area of 1.5 m². If the dosage is 0.2 g/m² and the form available is 125 mg/cc, how many cc will you administer? _____

SUMMARY OF CHAPTER 4 RULES

RULE 4.1   Rule for Metric Conversion

Step 1. Write the horizontal metric scale.

Step 2. Circle the two units stated in the problem.

Step 3. Count the number of metric units from the unit given to the unit desired. Note the direction.

Step 4. Move the decimal point the number of places counted in Step 3 and in the direction noted.

RULE 4.2   Conversion for the °F − °C Scales

$$\frac{°C}{°F - 32°} = \frac{5}{9}$$

RULE 4.3   Medication Rule

Ratio for medication on hand = Ratio for desired medication

(MOH = DM)

5
The Apothecaries' and Household Systems of Measurement and Conversions

OBJECTIVES

After studying this chapter you should be able to

1. read and write units in the apothecaries' and household systems of measurement;
2. convert from one unit of measure to another;
3. solve practical problems involving the apothecaries', household, and metric units of measure.

INTRODUCTION

The apothecaries' system of measurement is an ancient system that has been used by the medical profession for many years. (The word *apothecary* is derived from the Greek word meaning pharmacist.) The system was brought to the United States at the time of colonization, because it was part of the system used in England. Although the metric system is more accurate, the apothecaries' system is still used by some physicians when writing prescriptions and medication orders.

Roman numerals are used to state amounts in the apothecaries' system. These Roman numerals are written in lower case to the right of the apothecaries' unit of measure. Common fractions, except one-half, are written using Arabic numerals $\left(\text{for example, } \frac{1}{50}\right)$. One-half is written, $\overline{ss}$, which is an

100

abbreviation of the Latin word *semis,* meaning one-half. Decimals are not used for drug orders in the apothecaries' system. (For a review of Roman numerals, see Appendix I.)

5.1 APOTHECARIES' UNITS OF MEASURE

In the apothecaries' system of measurement, the basic unit of mass is the **grain**. When the system was established, the grain was defined as the average mass of a grain of wheat. The other units of mass in the apothecaries' system are the **dram** (ʒ), the **ounce** (℥), and the **pound** (lb). Their relationships are shown in Table 5–1.

TABLE 5–1 APOTHECARIES' UNITS OF MASS
60 grains (gr) = 1 dram (ʒ)
8 drams (ʒ) = 1 ounce (℥)
12 ounces (℥) = 1 pound (lb)

An apothecaries' pound is equal to 12 ℥. In our English system (avoirdupois system), a pound is equal to 16 oz. You should not confuse the two systems. The difference in these two systems arises from the definition of an ounce. In the apothecaries' system an oz is equivalent to 480 gr, while in the English system an oz is equal to 437.5 gr. The gr in both systems has the same mass.

The basic unit of volume in the apothecaries' system is the **minim** (𝔐). A 𝔐 is defined to be that volume of water that has the same mass as a grain of wheat. A 𝔐 is approximately equal to 1 drop of water.

The other units of volume in the apothecaries' system are the **fluid dram** (fʒ), the **fluid ounce** (f℥), **pint** (pt), **quart** (qt), and the **gallon** (gal). Their relationships are shown in Table 5–2.

TABLE 5–2 APOTHECARIES' UNITS OF VOLUME
60 minims (𝔐) = 1 fluid dram (fʒ)
8 fluid drams (fʒ) = 1 fluid ounce (f℥)
16 fluid ounces (f℥) = 1 pint (pt)
2 pints (pt) = 1 quart (qt)
4 quarts (qt) = 1 gallon (gal)

Medication orders and drug amounts may be written in the apothecaries' system using Rule 5.1.

> **RULE 5.1 Rule for Writing Measures in the Apothecaries' System**
>
> **Step 1.** Write the unit of measure in its abbreviated form.
>
> **Step 2.** Write the amount of the measure in Roman numeral form to the right of the apothecaries' abbreviated symbol.

EXAMPLE 5.1

Write each of the following measures in the apothecaries' abbreviated form.

(a) $6\frac{1}{2}$ fluid ounces

Step 1. The abbreviated form for fluid ounces is f℥. (Sometimes the *f* in f℥ is omitted when it is obvious that the medication is a liquid.)

Step 2. The Roman numeral for $6\frac{1}{2}$ = vi$\overline{\text{ss}}$.

Answer. $6\frac{1}{2}$ fluid ounces = f℥ vi$\overline{\text{ss}}$.

(b) 24 minims

Step 1. The abbreviated form for minim is ℳ.

Step 2. The Roman numeral for 24 is xxiv.

Answer. 24 minims = ℳ xxiv.

PRACTICE SET 5.1

Write each of the following measures in the apothecaries' abbreviated form.

1. 450 minims
2. 9 quarts
3. 1024 grains
4. 240 fluid drams
5. 764 ounces
6. 28 gallons
7. 906 fluid ounces
8. $88\frac{1}{2}$ drams

9. 43 ounces

10. 75 minims

11. 6 pints

12. $\dfrac{1}{50}$ grain

13. $2\dfrac{1}{2}$ fluid ounces

14. 59 pounds

15. 116 minims

16. 95 fluid drams

17. 17 ounces

18. $\dfrac{1}{250}$ grain

19. 4 gallons

20. 39 quarts

5.2 THE HOUSEHOLD UNITS OF MEASURE

The household system of measurement is the least accurate of the three systems of measurement. However, a household measure may be the only measure that a patient may have in the home.

There is no real basic unit of liquid measure in the household system, but the smallest unit used in the system is the **drop**. The abbreviation for drop is gtt, from the Latin word for drop, *gutta*. Not all drops are the same size. The size of a drop depends on the liquid's density and viscosity as well as on the size of the dropper opening. For practical purposes, however, a drop will be defined as a **minim**. Other units of measurement in the household system are stated in Table 5–3.

Household units are written using Arabic numerals. These numerals are written to the left of the abbreviated unit.

TABLE 5–3 HOUSEHOLD UNITS OF MEASUREMENT

75 drops (gtt) = 1 teaspoon (tsp)
3 teaspoons (tsp) = 1 tablespoon (tbsp)
2 tablespoons (tbsp) = 1 ounce (oz)
6 ounces (oz) = 1 teacup
8 ounces (oz) = 1 glass

EXAMPLE 5.2

Write each of the measures in the household abbreviated form.

(a) 415 drops

Answer. 415 gtt

(b) $5\frac{1}{2}$ ounces

Answer. $5\frac{1}{2}$ oz

PRACTICE SET 5.2

Write each of the following measures in the household abbreviated form.

1. 10 ounces
2. 150 drops
3. 5 tablespoons
4. 15 teaspoons
5. 35 ounces
6. 41 drops
7. 9 teaspoons
8. 12 tablespoons
9. 10 drops
10. 11 ounces

5.3 CONVERSIONS FROM ONE UNIT OF MEASURE TO ANOTHER

When using the apothecaries' or the household systems of measurement, it is sometimes necessary to convert from one unit to another. This can be done using Rule 5.2.

RULE 5.2 Conversion Rule

Step 1. Set up a conversion ratio from the table. (Include the unit labels in the ratio.)

Step 2. Set up a ratio from the problem. (Include the unit labels in the ratio.)

Step 3. Set the two ratios equal to each other.

Step 4. Solve for x.

5.3. Conversions from One Unit of Measure to Another

When setting the two ratios equal to each other, matched unit labels must appear in both the numerators and in both the denominators.

EXAMPLE 5.3

Change 3 ii$\overline{ss}$ to gr.

Step 1. Set up a conversion ratio from the table. To convert from ʒ to gr, a dram/grain ratio is needed. From the table, 60 gr = 1 ʒ. In ratio form, it is

$$\frac{60 \text{ gr}}{1 \text{ ʒ}}$$

Step 2. Set up a ratio from the problem. The problem asks how many gr are in $2\frac{1}{2}$ ʒ. The ratio is

$$\frac{x \text{ gr}}{2\frac{1}{2} \text{ ʒ}}$$

Step 3. Set the two ratios equal to each other.

$$\frac{60 \text{ gr}}{1 \text{ ʒ}} = \frac{x \text{ gr}}{2\frac{1}{2} \text{ ʒ}}$$

Check to see if the unit labels in both numerators and in both denominators agree.

Step 4. Solve for x.

Using the cross products rule:

$$\frac{60 \text{ gr}}{1 \text{ ʒ}} = \frac{x \text{ gr}}{2\frac{1}{2} \text{ ʒ}}$$

$$1x = (60)\left(2\frac{1}{2}\right)$$

$$x = 150$$

Answer. 3 ii$\overline{ss}$ = gr cl

In a proportion, Arabic numerals may be used to ease the calculations. The answer, however, should be written using Roman numerals and the abbreviated apothecaries' unit.

5. The Apothecaries' and Household Systems of Measurement and Conversions

EXAMPLE 5.4

Change f℥ xl to pt.

Step 1. Set up a conversion ratio from the table. To convert from f℥ to pt, an ounce-pint ratio is needed. From the table, 16 f℥ = 1 pt. In ratio form, it is

$$\frac{16 \text{ f℥}}{1 \text{ pt}}$$

Step 2. Set up a ratio from the problem. The problem asks how many pt in 40 f℥. The ratio is

$$\frac{40 \text{ f℥}}{x \text{ pt}}$$

Step 3. Set the two ratios equal to each other.

$$\frac{16 \text{ f℥}}{1 \text{ pt}} = \frac{40 \text{ f℥}}{x \text{ pt}}$$

Check to see if the unit labels agree in both numerators and in both denominators.

Step 4. Solve for x.

$$\frac{16 \text{ f℥}}{1 \text{ pt}} = \frac{40 \text{ f℥}}{x \text{ pt}}$$

$$16x = (40)(1)$$

$$x = 2\frac{1}{2} \text{ pt}$$

Answer. f℥ xl = pt iiss

EXAMPLE 5.5

Change ℥ ii to gr.

Set up a conversion ratio from the table. Since there is no direct conversion ratio from ℥ to gr, a plan should be devised.

Plan: ℥ ⟶ ℈ ⟶ gr
         Part 1   Part 2

Part 1.

Step 1. Since 1 ℥ = 8 ℈, the ratio is $\dfrac{1 \text{ ℥}}{8 \text{ ℈}}$.

5.3. Conversions from One Unit of Measure to Another

Step 2. From the problem, the ratio is $\dfrac{2\,\text{ʒ}}{x\,\text{ʒ}}$.

Step 3. $\qquad\qquad\qquad\qquad \dfrac{1\,\text{ʒ}}{8\,\text{ʒ}} = \dfrac{2\,\text{ʒ}}{x\,\text{ʒ}}$

Step 4. $\qquad\qquad\qquad\qquad \dfrac{1\,\text{ʒ}}{8\,\text{ʒ}} = \dfrac{2\,\text{ʒ}}{x\,\text{ʒ}}$

$$1x = (2)(8)$$
$$x = 16\,\text{ʒ}$$

Part 2. Change 16 ʒ to gr (take the answer from Part 1 and change it to gr).

Step 1. From the table, 1 ʒ = 60 gr. The ratio is

$$\dfrac{1\,\text{ʒ}}{60\,\text{gr}}$$

Step 2. From the problem, the ratio is

$$\dfrac{16\,\text{ʒ}}{x\,\text{gr}}$$

Step 3. $\qquad\qquad\qquad\qquad \dfrac{1\,\text{ʒ}}{60\,\text{gr}} = \dfrac{16\,\text{ʒ}}{x\,\text{gr}}$

$$1x = (16)(60)$$
$$x = 960\,\text{gr}$$

Answer.   ʒ ii = gr cmlx

EXAMPLE 5.6

Convert 28 oz to glasses.

Step 1. Set up a conversion ratio from the table.

$$8\,\text{oz} = 1\,\text{glass}$$

The ratio is

$$\dfrac{8\,\text{oz}}{1\,\text{glass}}$$

Step 2. Set up a ratio from the problem.

$$28\,\text{oz} = x\,\text{glasses}$$

The ratio is

$$\frac{28 \text{ oz}}{x \text{ glasses}}$$

Step 3. Set the ratios equal to each other.

$$\frac{8 \text{ oz}}{1 \text{ glass}} = \frac{28 \text{ oz}}{x \text{ glasses}}$$

Step 4. Solve for x.

$$\frac{8 \text{ oz}}{1 \text{ glass}} = \frac{28 \text{ oz}}{x \text{ glasses}}$$

$$8x = (28)(1)$$

$$x = 3\frac{1}{2} \text{ glasses}$$

Answer. 28 oz = $3\frac{1}{2}$ glasses

EXAMPLE 5.7

Change 8 oz to tsp.

This example implies two parts, since there is no direct conversion from oz to tsp.

Plan. 8 oz $\longrightarrow$ tbsp $\longrightarrow$ tsp
            ___Part 1___   __Part 2__

Part 1. Change 8 oz to tbsp.

Step 1. Since 1 oz = 2 tbsp, the ratio is

$$\frac{1 \text{ oz}}{2 \text{ tbsp}}$$

Step 2. From the problem, the ratio is

$$\frac{8 \text{ oz}}{x \text{ tbsp}}$$

Step 3. $\quad\dfrac{1 \text{ oz}}{2 \text{ tbsp}} = \dfrac{8 \text{ oz}}{x \text{ tbsp}}$

Step 4. $\quad x = 16 \text{ tbsp}$

5.3. Conversions from One Unit of Measure to Another   109

Part 2. Change 16 tbsp to tsp (using the answer from Part 1).

Step 1. From the table, 3 tsp = 1 tbsp, so the ratio is

$$\frac{3 \text{ tsp}}{1 \text{ tbsp}}$$

Step 2. From the problem, the ratio is

$$\frac{x \text{ tsp}}{16 \text{ tbsp}}$$

Step 3. $\frac{3 \text{ tsp}}{1 \text{ tbsp}} = \frac{x \text{ tsp}}{16 \text{ tbsp}}$

$$1x = (3)(16)$$

Step 4. $x = 48$ tsp

Answer. 8 oz = 48 tsp

PRACTICE SET 5.3

Change each of the following units to the indicated unit.

1. ʒ xxxvi = ℥ _____
2. pt s̄s̄ = ℳ _____
3. fʒ xxxii = qt _____
4. ℳ cl = fʒ _____
5. gr mcdxl = ℥ _____
6. fʒ iv = ℳ _____
7. gal s̄s̄ = pt _____
8. qt xii = fʒ _____
9. ℳ mmcd = fʒ _____
10. fʒ $\frac{1}{8}$ = fʒ _____
11. Change 150 gtt to tsp.
12. Change 44 oz to glasses.
13. Change 1 tbsp to oz.
14. Change 2 ounces to gtt.
15. Change 5 glasses to tbsp.
16. 3600 gtt = _____ tbsp
17. 4.5 tbsp = _____ tsp
18. 76 tbsp = _____ glasses
19. 3 oz = _____ tsp
20. $1\frac{1}{2}$ tsp = _____ gtt

5.4 APPLICATIONS INVOLVING APOTHECARIES', HOUSEHOLD, AND METRIC UNITS

A comparison of the triple systems of measurement is shown on the medicine glass in Figure 5–1.

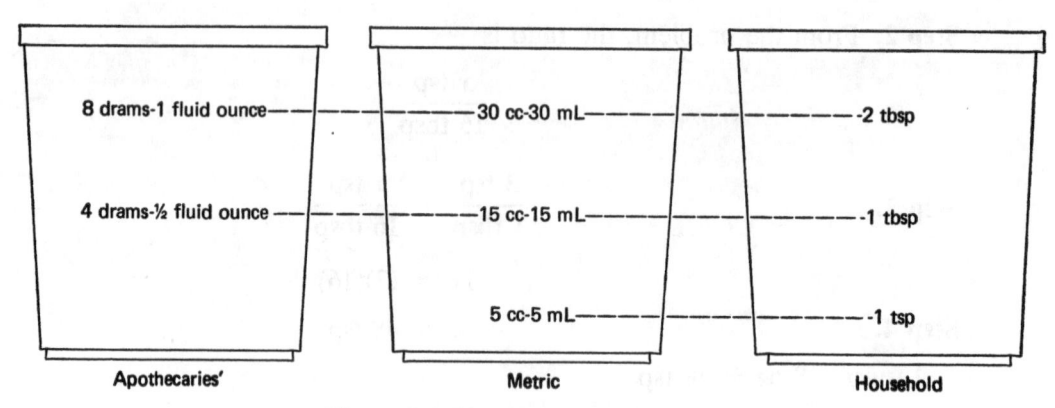

```
Apothecaries':  8 drams-1 fluid ounce
                4 drams-½ fluid ounce
Metric:         30 cc-30 mL
                15 cc-15 mL
                5 cc-5 mL
Household:      -2 tbsp
                -1 tbsp
                -1 tsp
```

Figure 5–1 The medicine glass.

You should be able to convert from one system of measurement to another. Table 5–4 shows approximate equivalents needed to perform these conversions. It is imperative that you memorize this table.

Rule 5.2 can be used to perform the conversions from one system to another.

EXAMPLE 5.8

Convert 18 mL to tsp.

Step 1. $\dfrac{5 \text{ mL}}{1 \text{ tsp}}$ (Conversion ratio from the table)

Step 2. $\dfrac{18 \text{ mL}}{x \text{ tsp}}$ (Ratio from the problem)

Steps 3–4.
$$\frac{5 \text{ mL}}{1 \text{ tsp}} = \frac{18 \text{ mL}}{x \text{ tsp}}$$
$$5x = 18$$
$$x = 3\frac{3}{5} \text{ tsp}$$

Answer. $18 \text{ mL} = 3\dfrac{3}{5} \text{ tsp}$.

5.4. Applications Involving Apothecaries', Household, and Metric Units

TABLE 5–4 TABLE OF APPROXIMATE EQUIVALENTS

Household	Apothecaries'	Metric
	Mass	
	1 gr	60 mg (60–65)*
	$1\frac{1}{2}$ gr	100 mg
	15 gr	1 g
	60 gr = 1 ʒ	4 g
	8 ʒ = 1 ℥	30 g
2.2 lb		1 kg
	Volume	
15 gtt	15 ℳ (15–16)	1 mL (1 cc)
60 gtt	1 f ʒ	4 mL
1 tsp (75 gtt)	$\frac{1}{6}$ f ʒ	5 mL
1 tbsp (3 tsp)	$\frac{1}{2}$ f ʒ	15 mL
2 tbsp	1 f ℥	30 mL (30–32)
16 oz	1 pt	500 mL
1 qt	1 qt	1000 mL (1 L)
1 glass	8 fluid ounces	
	Length	
39.4 in.		1 m
1 in.		2.54 cm

*Note that a range of values is given for several equivalents. This range is necessary because of the approximate values of the apothecaries' system. For discussions in this book, the first mentioned value will be used for a consistency of answers. Other books may use other values within the range.

EXAMPLE 5.9

A patient weighs 120 kg. How many lb is this?

Using the proportion:

$$\frac{1 \text{ kg}}{2.2 \text{ lb}} = \frac{120 \text{ kg}}{x \text{ lb}}$$

$$1x = (120)(2.2)$$

$$x = 264 \text{ lb}$$

Answer. The patient weighs 264 lb.

5. The Apothecaries' and Household Systems of Measurement and Conversions

Often the apothecaries' system is used in medication problems such as those shown in Chapter 3.

EXAMPLE 5.10

A liquid medicine has gr $\overline{ss}$ drug dissolved in f℥ i. Administer gr $\frac{1}{4}$. How many drams should be given?

$$\text{MOH} = \text{DM}$$
$$\frac{\frac{1}{2}\text{gr}}{1\,\mathfrak{Z}} = \frac{\frac{1}{4}\text{gr}}{x\,\mathfrak{Z}}$$

$$\frac{1}{2}x = \left(\frac{1}{4}\right)(1)$$

$$\frac{1}{2}x = \frac{1}{4}$$

$$\left(\frac{2}{1}\right)\frac{1}{2}x = \left(\frac{2}{1}\right)\left(\frac{1}{4}\right)$$

$$x = \frac{1}{2}$$

Answer. Administer ℨ $\overline{ss}$ of the liquid medicine.

EXAMPLE 5.11

A syrup has gr $\frac{1}{6}$ dissolved in f℥ ii; give gr $\frac{1}{8}$. How many 𝔐 should you give? Divide this problem into two parts. In Part 1 find the number of ℨ in which gr $\frac{1}{8}$ is dissolved. Then in Part 2 convert the ℨ to 𝔐.

Part 1. Calculate desired medication.

$$\text{MOH} = \text{DM}$$
$$\frac{\frac{1}{6}\text{gr}}{2\,\mathfrak{Z}} = \frac{\frac{1}{8}\text{gr}}{x\,\mathfrak{Z}}$$

5.4. Applications Involving Apothecaries', Household, and Metric Units

$$\frac{1}{6}x = \left(\frac{1}{8}\right)(2)$$

$$\frac{1}{6}x = \frac{2}{8}$$

$$\left(\frac{6}{1}\right)\frac{1}{6}x = \left(\frac{6}{1}\right)\left(\frac{2}{8}\right)$$

$$x = \frac{12}{8}$$

$$x = 1\frac{1}{2} ʒ$$

Part 2. Convert $1\frac{1}{2}$ ʒ to ℳ.

Step 1. Ratio from table is

$$\frac{60 \; ℳ}{1 \; ʒ}$$

Step 2. Ratio from problem is

$$\frac{x \; ℳ}{1\frac{1}{2} \; ʒ}$$

Step 3.
$$\frac{60 \; ℳ}{1 \; ʒ} = \frac{x \; ℳ}{1\frac{1}{2} \; ʒ}$$

Step 4.
$$1x = (60)\left(1\frac{1}{2}\right)$$

$$x = 90$$

Answer. Administer ℳ xc of the syrup to the patient.

EXAMPLE 5.12

Medication on hand: gr $2\frac{3}{4}$ tabs. Order: gr v̄s̄s̄. How many tabs should be administered?

$$MOH = DM$$

$$\frac{2\frac{3}{4} \text{ gr}}{1 \text{ tab}} = \frac{5\frac{1}{2} \text{ gr}}{x \text{ tabs}}$$

$$2\frac{3}{4}x = \left(5\frac{1}{2}\right)(1)$$

$$\left(\frac{4}{11}\right)\frac{11}{4}x = \left(\frac{4}{11}\right)\frac{11}{2}$$

$$x = 2 \text{ tabs}$$

Answer. Administer 2 tabs $\left(\text{gr } 2\frac{3}{4}/\text{tab}\right)$

EXAMPLE 5.13

A magnesium sulfate solution 0.2 mL/kg body mass is prescribed by a physician. How many mL will a 160 lb patient receive?

Divide this problem into two parts. In Part 1, pounds should be converted to kg; and in Part 2, the desired medication should be calculated.

Part 1. Convert pounds to kg.

$$\frac{1 \text{ kg}}{2.2 \text{ lb}} = \frac{x \text{ kg}}{160 \text{ lb}}$$

$$2.2x = 160$$

$$x = 72.73 \text{ kg}$$

Part 2. Calculate desired medication.

$$MOH = DM$$

$$\frac{0.2 \text{ mL}}{1 \text{ kg}} = \frac{x \text{ mL}}{72.73 \text{ kg}}$$

$$1x = (0.2)(72.73)$$

$$x = 14.5 \text{ mL}$$

Answer. Administer 14.5 mL to the patient.

5.4. Applications Involving Apothecaries', Household, and Metric Units

EXAMPLE 5.14

A prescription calls for a dose of 3 tsp of Oxaine to be administered 4 times each day, 15 minutes before meals and at bedtime. How many days will a 350 mL bottle of Oxaine last?

Divide this problem into three parts. In Part 1, find the number of mL in 3 tsp; in Part 2, find the number of mL to be administered per day; and in Part 3, find the number of days the 350 mL bottle will last.

Part 1. Convert 3 tsp to mL.

$$\frac{1 \text{ tsp}}{5 \text{ mL}} = \frac{3 \text{ tsp}}{x \text{ mL}}$$

$$1x = (3)(5)$$

$$x = 15 \text{ mL}$$

Part 2. Calculate number of mL per day.

$$15 \text{ mL} \times 4 \text{ times per day} = 60 \text{ mL/day}$$

Part 3. Find the number of days bottle will last.

$$350 \text{ mL} \div 60 \text{ mL/day} = 5.8 \text{ days}$$

Answer. The 350 mL will last 5 days; there is not enough for 6 days.

EXAMPLE 5.15

Phenobarbital suppositories in doses of 8 mg, 15 mg, 30 mg, 60 mg, .1 g, and .12 g are available in the pharmacy. Which will you order to administer the following:

(a) gr $\overline{\text{ss}}$

Convert gr $\overline{\text{ss}}$ to mg and then choose the correct suppository size.

$$\frac{1 \text{ gr}}{60 \text{ mg}} = \frac{\frac{1}{2} \text{ gr}}{x \text{ mg}}$$

$$1x = \left(\frac{1}{2}\right)(60)$$

$$x = 30 \text{ mg}$$

Answer. Order a 30 mg phenobarbital suppository for gr $\overline{\text{ss}}$.

(b) gr ii

$$\frac{1 \text{ gr}}{60 \text{ mg}} = \frac{2 \text{ gr}}{x \text{ mg}}$$

$$1x = (2)(60)$$

$$x = 120 \text{ mg}$$

There is no 120 mg suppository listed. Therefore, convert 120 mg to grams and compare the suppositories.

$$120 \text{ mg} = 0.12 \text{ g}$$

Answer. Order the 0.12 g phenobarbital suppository for gr ii.

EXAMPLE 5.16

A mother is instructed to give her child 2 oz of cough syrup divided into two equal doses. How many tbsp is this?

$$\frac{1 \text{ oz}}{2 \text{ tbsp}} = \frac{2 \text{ oz}}{x \text{ tbsp}}$$

$$x = (2)(2)$$

$$x = 4 \text{ tbsp}$$

Answer. The child should receive 4 tbsp of cough syrup in two equally divided doses.

EXAMPLE 5.17

If a patient drinks 3 glasses of water and 1 glass of orange juice during 1 day, how many oz of liquid has the patient consumed?

Total amount of liquid in 4 glasses:

$$\frac{1 \text{ glass}}{8 \text{ oz}} = \frac{4 \text{ glasses}}{x \text{ oz}}$$

$$x = (4)(8)$$

$$x = 32 \text{ oz}$$

Answer. The patient has consumed 32 oz of liquid.

EXAMPLE 5.18

How would you advise a patient to administer the following dosages in the home?

(a) 5 mg of a drug, if the drug is available in 2.5 mg/cc.

5.4. Applications Involving Apothecaries', Household, and Metric Units

Usually a patient is familiar with a tsp, tbsp, and an oz. Therefore, convert the above medication to one of these units.

Part 1. Calculate the desired medication.

$$\underset{\downarrow}{\text{MOH}} = \underset{\downarrow}{\text{DM}}$$

$$\frac{2.5 \text{ mg}}{1 \text{ cc}} = \frac{5 \text{ mg}}{x \text{ cc}}$$

$$2.5x = (5)(1)$$

$$x = 2 \text{ cc}$$

Part 2. Convert 2 cc to a tsp (a common household measure).

$$\frac{1 \text{ tsp}}{5 \text{ cc}} = \frac{x \text{ tsp}}{2 \text{ cc}}$$

$$5x = (2)(1)$$

$$x = \frac{2}{5}$$

Answer. $\frac{2}{5}$ is approximately $\frac{1}{2}$; therefore, administer about $\frac{1}{2}$ tsp of the medicine.

(b) 3 ʒ Pepto-Bismol.

Plan. Change $\underbrace{\text{ʒ} \longrightarrow \text{mL}}_{\text{Part 1}} \underbrace{\longrightarrow \text{tsp}}_{\text{Part 2}}$

Part 1. Convert drams to mL.

$$\frac{1 \text{ ʒ}}{4 \text{ mL}} = \frac{3 \text{ ʒ}}{x \text{ mL}}$$

$$1x = (3)(4)$$

$$x = 12 \text{ mL}$$

Part 2. Convert mL to tsp.

$$\frac{1 \text{ tsp}}{5 \text{ mL}} = \frac{x \text{ tsp}}{12 \text{ mL}}$$

$$5x = (12)(1)$$

$$x = 2\frac{2}{5} \approx 2\frac{1}{2} \text{ tsp}$$

Answer. Patient should take about $2\frac{1}{2}$ tsp Pepto-Bismol.

EXAMPLE 5.19

If the human ovum is about 0.14 mm in diameter, what is this diameter expressed in inches? Round off to the nearest thousandth.

Plan. Convert mm $\longrightarrow$ cm $\longrightarrow$ in.
              Part 1   Part 2

Part 1. Convert 0.14 mm to cm.

$$0.14 \text{ mm} = 0.014 \text{ cm}$$

Part 2. Convert 0.014 cm to in.

$$\frac{2.54 \text{ cm}}{1 \text{ in.}} = \frac{0.014 \text{ cm}}{x \text{ in.}}$$

$$2.54x = (1)(0.014)$$

$$x = 0.0055 \text{ in.} \approx 0.006 \text{ in.}$$

Answer. The human ovum is approximately 0.006 in. in diameter.

PRACTICE SET 5.4

1. Convert 13.8 cm to in.
2. Convert 7.5 cc to ℳ.
3. Convert gr $\frac{3}{4}$ to mg.
4. Convert 15 kg to lb.
5. Convert 4 tbsp to mL.
6. Convert gr viiss to g.
7. Convert $412\frac{1}{2}$ gtt to tsp.
8. Convert ʒ ii to tbsp.
9. Drug order: atropine gr $\frac{1}{200}$. The available form is gr $\frac{1}{150}$/cc. How many cc should be administered?

5.5. Chapter 5 Review Problems

10. An injectable liquid has gr $\frac{1}{150}$ in ℳ x. The drug order calls for gr $\frac{1}{250}$. How many minims should be given?

11. If a patient drinks 3 glasses of fluid, how many oz has she consumed?

12. If a patient is to take 1 oz of Milk of Magnesia at home, what household measure can she use other than an oz glass?

13. Order: gr $\frac{1}{200}$.

    Medication on hand: gr $\frac{1}{100}$ scored tablets.

    How many tabs should be administered?

14. A patient is to receive 1 tbsp per dose of a particular medicine. How many doses will a 3-oz bottle contain?

15. A capsule contains gr iv of a drug. How many ʒ of this drug will be contained in 60 capsules?

16. Drug order: aspirin gr x.
    Form available: aspirin 600 mg tab.
    How many tablets should be used?

17. Drug order: morphine gr $\frac{1}{4}$.

    Form available: 5 mL vial of morphine, 10 mg/mL.
    How many mL of morphine should be administered?

18. A patient has been prescribed 30 mL of Milk of Magnesia. What household measure should she use, and how much of it?

19. A physician prescribes epinephrine for a patient, 0.1 mL/kg body mass. How much will a 77-lb patient receive?

20. A drug is to be administered to a 187-lb patient. The order calls for 50 mg/kg body mass. The drug is to be administered in two equally divided doses. How many g per dose should be administered?

5.5 CHAPTER 5 REVIEW PROBLEMS

Write out the following using Arabic numerals.

1. ʒ cdxxiv _____
2. pt lxix$\overline{\overline{ss}}$ _____

120   5.   The Apothecaries' and Household Systems of Measurement and Conversions

3. gr xxviiss _____
4. lb mdlx _____
5. gal lxxii _____

Abbreviate the following using the apothecaries' system.

6. 412 fluid drams _____
7. 725 minims _____
8. $80\frac{1}{2}$ pints _____
9. 42 quarts _____
10. 1140 grains _____
11. 221 ounces _____

Complete each of the following:

12. ʒ iss = gr _____
13. gr cl = ʒ _____
14. ʒ xxxii = ℥ _____
15. pt iss = ℥ _____
16. 2 tbsp = _____ gtt
17. 20 oz = _____ tbsp
18. 6 oz = _____ glasses
19. $\frac{1}{8}$ glass = _____ tbsp
20. 27 tsp = _____ tbsp
21. ʒ ss = ℳ _____
22. ʒ ivss = ʒ _____
23. ℳ ccxl = ʒ _____
24. Convert 40 cc to ℳ.
25. Convert 15 pt to mL.
26. Convert 225 gr to g.
27. Convert 18 kg to lb.

5.5. Chapter 5 Review Problems

28. Convert 18 cc to f♂.

29. Convert 60 gtt to 𝔐.

30. Convert f♂ xxiv to tbsp.

31. Convert 44 oz to glasses.

32. Convert $5\frac{1}{2}$ qt to L.

33. If the large intestine is approximately $1\frac{1}{2}$ m long, about how many in. is this?

Solve the following problems.

34. You are to give morphine sulfate gr $\frac{1}{8}$ from a solution of morphine sulfate labeled gr $\frac{1}{12}$: 𝔐 xvi. How many 𝔐 will you give?

35. If a capsule contains gr v of a drug, how many ♂ of this drug would be required to make up 60 capsules?

36. A vial is labeled gr $\frac{1}{10}$ / 𝔐 xxxv. Administer gr $\frac{1}{25}$. How many 𝔐 will you administer?

37. A physician orders gr iss of Seconal medication. You have capsules containing gr $\frac{3}{4}$. How many capsules should you give?

38. You are to administer f♂ i of a particular medication. How many doses will a f♂ iv bottle contain?

39. You are to give gr ivss of aspirin. You have capsules containing gr iss and gr i. How many of which capsule should you give?

40. Desired dose: gr $\frac{1}{50}$: Medication on hand: gr $\frac{1}{400}$ tabs. How many tabs will you give?

41. Desired medication: gr xv: Medication on hand: gr viiss/tab. How many tabs will you give?

42. A vial on hand is labeled gr $\frac{1}{4}$: 𝔐 xx. Give gr $\frac{1}{8}$. How many 𝔐 will you administer?

43. A doctor prescribes ℳ x of Lugol's solution per dose for a patient. A ʒ ii bottle of Lugol's solution is on hand. How many doses does the bottle contain?

44. If a patient drinks 28 oz of water and 12 oz of juice during the course of 1 day, how many glasses did the patient consume?

45. If a patient is to take $1\frac{1}{2}$ oz of Milk of Magnesia, how many tbsp should the patient take?

46. A patient is to receive $\frac{1}{2}$ tbsp per dose of a particular medicine 3 times per day. How many days will a 2-oz bottle last?

47. A patient takes 2 tbsp of a cough syrup three times a day. How many tsp does the patient take each day?

48. Sodium benzoate is available 250 mg/mL. How many mL will you administer if the doctor's order calls for gr viii?

49. How would you advise a patient to take 6 mg of hydrocodone bitartrate at home if the hydrocodone bitartrate label reads 2.5 mg/mL?

50. Sulfathiazole, a cream, has been prescribed for a patient having a vaginal infection. If the cream comes in a 75 g tube, how many oz does the tube contain?

5.6 CHAPTER 5 SELF TEST

Convert each unit as indicated.

5.1 5.3	1. ʒ viss = gr	_____	
5.1 5.3	2. fʒ xiv =	_____	mL
5.1 5.3	3. fʒ $\frac{1}{4}$ = fʒ	_____	
5.1 5.3	4. pt xxviii = fʒ	_____	
5.3	5. 135 mL =	_____	oz
5.2 5.3	6. 5 tbsp =	_____	gtt
5.2 5.3	7. 28 oz =	_____	tsp

Summary of Chapter 5 Rules

5.2 5.3   **8.** 14 oz = _____ glasses

5.3   **9.** gr $\dfrac{1}{150}$ = _____ mg

5.1 5.3   **10.** 4 mL = ℳ _____

Solve. Be sure to label all your answers.

5.1   **11.** Drug order: Digoxin gr $\dfrac{1}{300}$. Available form: gr $\dfrac{1}{150}$ scored tabs. How many tabs should you give? _____

5.4   **12.** A doctor prescribes 10 cc of Milk of Magnesia for a patient. What household measurement would you advise the patient to use, and how much of it? _____

5.4   **13.** Order: Phenobarbital gr $\overline{ss}$.
Medication on hand: 15 mg, 30 mg, 60 mg tabs.
How many tabs of which strength should you administer? _____

5.4   **14.** Nembutal is available as gr $\overline{iss}$/tab. A doctor prescribes gr ix total in three equally divided doses. How many tabs will you give per dose? _____

5.4   **15.** A doctor prescribes meperidine hydrochloride 6000 mcg/kg body mass total daily in four equally divided doses for a patient weighing 77 lb. How many mg should be administered per dose? _____

SUMMARY OF CHAPTER 5 RULES

RULE 5.1   Rule for Writing Measures in the Apothecaries' System

Step 1. Write the unit of measure in its abbreviated form.

Step 2. Write the amount of the measure in Roman numeral form to the right of the apothecaries' abbreviated symbol.

RULE 5.2 Conversion Rule

Step 1. Set up a conversion ratio from the table. (Include the unit labels in the ratio.)

Step 2. Set up a ratio from the problem. (Include the unit labels in the ratio.)

Step 3. Set the two ratios equal to each other.

Step 4. Solve for x.

6
Calculations for Oral and Parenteral Dosages

OBJECTIVES

After studying this chapter you should be able to

1. calculate dosages of tablets and capsules;
2. calculate dosages of oral solutions;
3. calculate dosages of injectable drugs.

INTRODUCTION

Oral administration of drugs is one of the most common methods of administering drugs to patients. Not only are oral drugs easy to take, but they are also very convenient and economical. Since they are absorbed through the gastrointestinal tract, the skin is not broken, thus minimizing the danger of infection through interrupted skin.

A physician prescribes the drug order for a patient. In so doing, the physician generally uses medical abbreviations, a type of shorthand that has become the international language of professionals concerned with patient care. This shorthand writing uses Latin abbreviations. If you are not familiar with these medical abbreviations, study Appendix II. These abbreviations must be memorized.

Once the drug order is written, you may have to obtain the medication, prepare it, and administer it. Many hospitals have unit dosages already prepared by the manufacturer. Thus, most dosages may be obtained in the required dosage form. However, if a certain drug is not prepared in the strength prescribed by the physician, you should be able to calculate the correct dosage.

6.1 CALCULATING DOSAGES OF TABLETS AND CAPSULES

Some of the most common forms of drugs are tablets and capsules. Some tablets are scored for easy division into parts; unscored tablets and capsules must never be divided. Tablets come in different strengths, expressed in either metric measures, apothecaries' measures, milliequivalents, or units. Examples of these are: Nembutal 100 mg capsules, Proloid $\frac{1}{2}$ gr tablets, V-Cillin K 400 000 unit tablets, and potassium chloride 20 milliequivalent tablets.

You are already familiar with the metric and apothecaries' measures. Another drug measure, the **unit** (U) is based on weight and is defined in terms of the effect that the specific drug has on the body. For example, a unit of penicillin is standardized according to its ability to lower bacterial activity; a unit of insulin is measured according to its ability to lower sugar in the bloodstream.

A **milliequivalent** (mEq), on the other hand, is defined in terms of its combining power instead of its weight. In general, one milliequivalent is said to have the same chemical combining power as 1 mg of hydrogen.

Use Rule 6.1 to calculate the correct dosage of tablets or capsules. This rule has already been used in Chapter 3.

RULE 6.1 Rule for Calculating Tablet and Capsule Dosage

Step 1. Write the medication on hand (MOH) as a ratio.

Step 2. Write the desired medication (DM) as a ratio.

Step 3. Set the two ratios equal to each other and solve for x.

EXAMPLE 6.1

Order: Gantrisin gr xxv.
Medication on hand: Gantrisin 500 mg tabs.
How many tabs will you administer to the patient?
Using Rule 6.1:

$$\underset{\downarrow}{\text{MOH}} = \underset{\downarrow}{\text{DM}}$$

$$\frac{500 \text{ mg}}{1 \text{ tab}} = \frac{25 \text{ gr}}{x \text{ tab}}$$

The numerators must have like units. Since 1 gr = 60 mg, 25 gr = 1500 mg. By substitution:

6.1. Calculating Dosages of Tablets and Capsules

$$\begin{array}{c} \text{MOH} = \text{DM} \\ \downarrow \quad\quad \downarrow \\ \dfrac{500 \text{ mg}}{1 \text{ tab}} = \dfrac{1500 \text{ mg}}{x \text{ tabs}} \leftarrow 25 \text{ gr} \end{array}$$

$$500x = (1500)(1)$$

$$x = 3$$

Answer. Administer 3 tabs of Gantrisin (500 mg/tab).

EXAMPLE 6.2

Determine the number of tabs necessary to administer the correct dosage for the following prescription (Fig. 6–1).

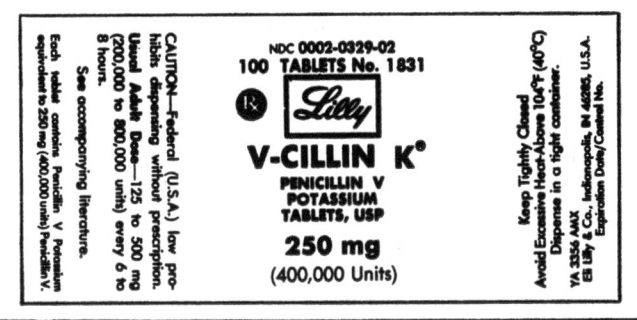

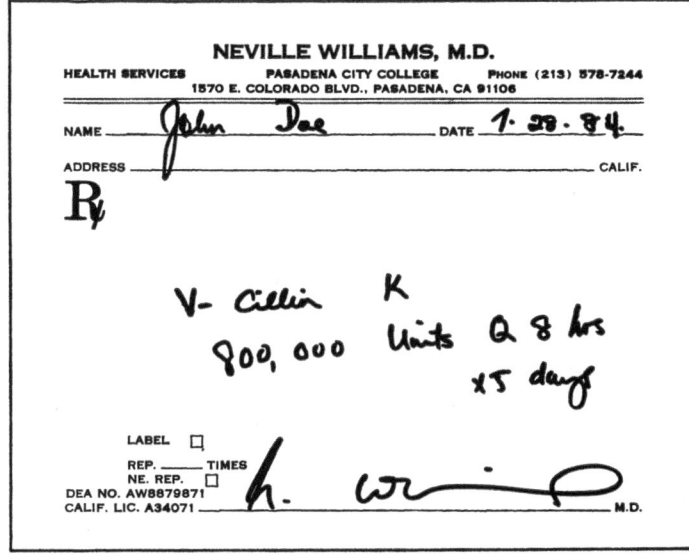

Figure 6–1. V-Cillin K and prescription

$$\text{MOH} = \text{DM}$$
$$\frac{400\ 000\ \text{U}}{1\ \text{tab}} = \frac{800\ 000\ \text{U}}{x\ \text{tabs}}$$
$$400\ 000x = 800\ 000$$
$$x = 2$$

Answer. Give John Doe 2 tabs/dose of V-Cillin K (400 000 U/tab).

EXAMPLE 6.3

An order is for 2 500 000 units of penicillin G potassium daily in two equally divided doses. Penicillin G potassium is available in 100 000 unit tabs, 250 000 unit tabs, and 500 000 unit tabs. Which strength tabs should be used and how many should the patient receive?

Divide this problem into two parts.

Part 1. Calculate the amount of penicillin G per dose.

$$2\ 500\ 000\ \text{U} \div 2\ \text{doses} = 1\ 250\ 000\ \text{U/dose}$$

Part 2. Calculate the number of tabs per dose. Since it is best to use the least number of tabs, use the penicillin tab of greatest strength for the calculation.

Greatest strength tab →
$$\frac{500\ 000\ \text{U}}{1\ \text{tab}} = \frac{1\ 250\ 000\ \text{U}}{x\ \text{tabs}}$$
$$500\ 000x = 1\ 250\ 000$$
$$x = 2\tfrac{1}{2}\ \text{tabs of 500 000 U}$$

Since these penicillin G tabs are not scored, they cannot be divided. Another tab equal to $\tfrac{1}{2}$ of 500 000 U must be selected.

$$\tfrac{1}{2}\ \text{of 500 000 U} = 250\ 000$$

Use a 250 000 U tab.

Answer. Administer 2 tabs of 500 000 U and 1 tab of 250 000 U penicillin G.

EXAMPLE 6.4

Order: 50 000 units of penicillin G potassium per kg body mass per day, to be administered in four equally divided doses. Penicillin G potassium 500 000 unit tabs are available. How many tabs will a 176-lb patient receive?

6.1. Calculating Dosages of Tablets and Capsules

Divide this problem into four parts:

Part 1. Change 176 lb to kg.

$$\frac{2.2 \text{ lb}}{1 \text{ kg}} = \frac{176 \text{ lb}}{x \text{ kg}}$$

$$2.2x = (176)(1)$$

$$x = 80 \text{ kg}$$

The patient weighs 80 kg.

Part 2. If the prescribed dosage is 50 000 U/kg, calculate the amount of penicillin for this 80-kg patient.

$$\frac{50\ 000 \text{ U}}{1 \text{ kg}} = \frac{x \text{ U}}{80 \text{ kg}}$$

$$x = (50\ 000)(80)$$

$$x = 4\ 000\ 000 \text{ U}$$

Part 3. Calculate units per dose.

$$4\ 000\ 000 \text{ U} \div 4 \text{ doses} = 1\ 000\ 000 \text{ U}$$

Part 4. Calculate desired medication.

$$\frac{\overset{\text{MOH}}{\downarrow}}{500\ 000 \text{ U}} = \frac{\overset{\text{DM}}{\downarrow}}{1\ 000\ 000 \text{ U}}$$
$$\frac{500\ 000 \text{ U}}{1 \text{ tab}} = \frac{1\ 000\ 000 \text{ U}}{x \text{ tabs}}$$

$$500\ 000x = (1)(1\ 000\ 000)$$

$$x = 2 \text{ tabs}$$

Answer. Administer 2 tabs of penicillin G potassium 500 000 U/tab per dose.

PRACTICE SET 6.1

1. Order: Colace 0.25 g po qd.
   Medication on hand: Colace 50 mg capsules.
   How many capsules should be administered to the patient?

2. How many mg of potassium chloride will John Doe receive each dose? Use the drug label and Dr. Williams' prescription to calculate the correct amount (Fig. 6–2).

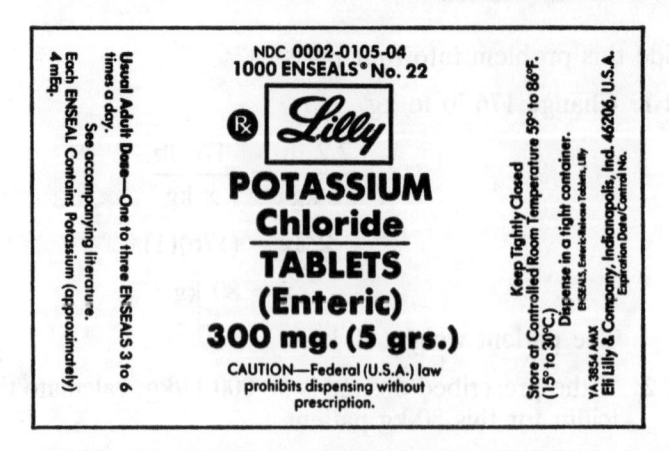

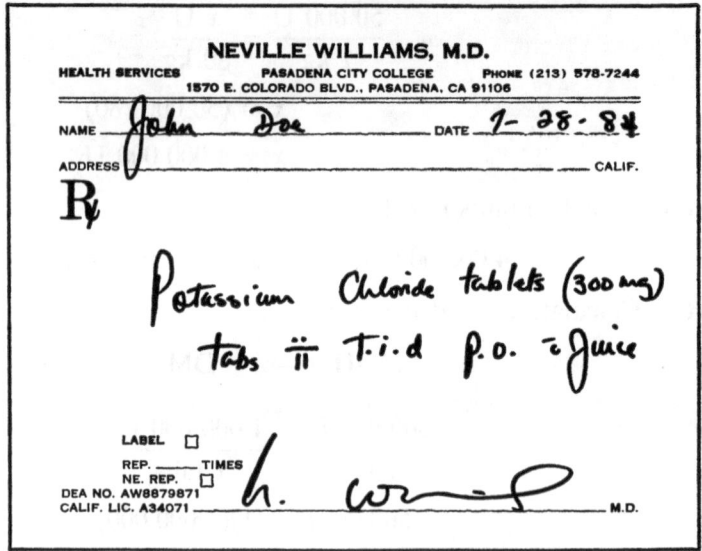

Figure 6–2. Potassium chloride and prescription

3. Order: 650 mg po stat (Fig. 6–3). How many tabs should be administered?

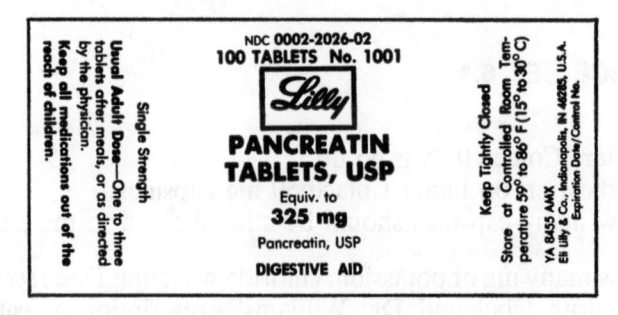

6.1. Calculating Dosages of Tablets and Capsules

4. A patient is suffering from a severe infection. The physician prescribes 1000 mg Tegopen po q6h for the infection. Tegopen is available in the pharmacy as 250 mg tabs. How many tablets should the patient take per dose?

5. Achromycin-V is available as a 250 mg capsule. Achromycin-V 0.5 g po qid is ordered for a patient. How many capsules should be administered per dose?

6. Calculate the correct number of tabs of phenobarbital per dose for this patient (Fig. 6–4).

7. Order: Tylenol gr x po q3h.
   Available: Tylenol 300 mg tabs.
   How many tabs per dose should be administered?

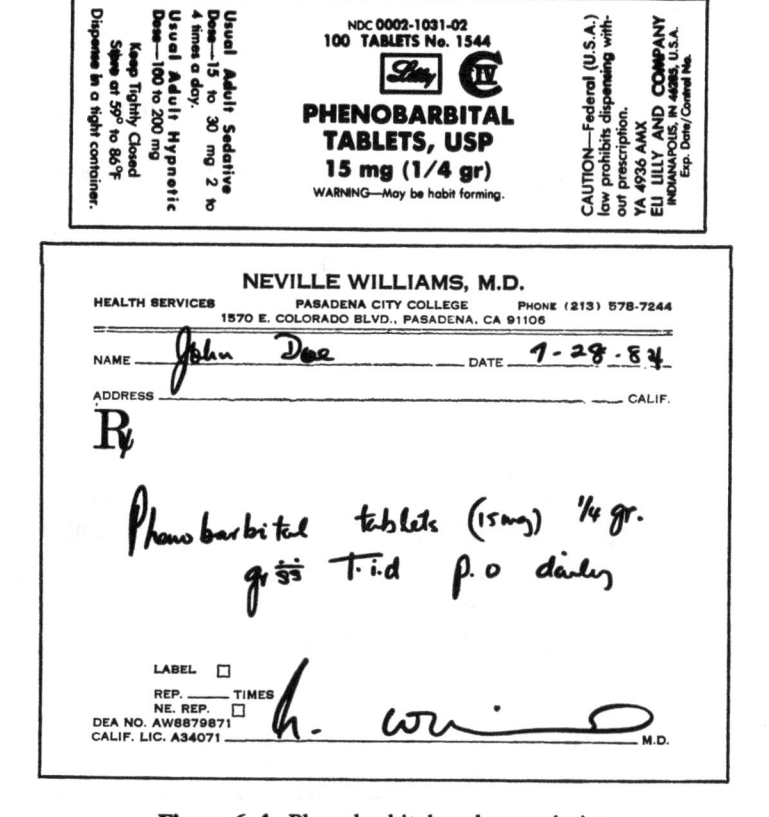

Figure 6–4. Phenobarbital and prescription

8. An order is for codeine 40 mg prn. The drug label reads codeine gr $\frac{1}{3}$/tab. How many tabs should be administered prn?

9. An order is for 3 000 000 units of penicillin G potassium daily in two equally divided doses. The available forms of penicillin G potassium are 100 000 U/tab, 150 000 U/tab, and 500 000 U/tab. Which strength tabs should be used, and how many should be administered?

10. Order: 30 000 units of penicillin G potassium per kg body mass per day to be administered in three equally divided doses. Tablets available are 100 000 unit scored tabs. How many tabs will a 110-lb patient receive per dose?

6.2 CALCULATING DOSAGES OF ORAL SOLUTIONS

Some patients find it difficult to swallow capsules or tablets. Therefore, many drugs are available in an oral solution or in the form of a powder to be reconstituted as a liquid.

Since some drugs are unstable in liquid form, they are packaged in powdered form in sterile ampules or vials. A powdered drug alone may have an expiration date of 2 to 5 years, while a reconstituted liquid drug may last only 10 to 14 days. Therefore, a powdered drug form is not reconstituted until its actual use is required.

Directions for dissolving powdered drugs will always be found on the label of the vial or ampule or in the accompanying literature. These directions will generally state the type and amount of solvent to be used. It will also state the resulting solution's strength; that is, the amount of drug per amount of solution.

To calculate the correct dosage of an oral solution for a patient, use Rule 6.1.

EXAMPLE 6.5

Calculate the amount of chloral hydrate elixir to be administered.

Drug Order		Drug Label
Name	J. Jones	Chloral hydrate elixir
Room	201	
Drug	Chloral hydrate elixir	gr $\overline{\text{viiss}}$/5 mL
Dose	500 mg	
Route	po	
Time	hs	

6.2. Calculating Dosages of Oral Solutions

Using Rule 6.1:

$$\frac{\overset{\downarrow}{MOH}}{5 \text{ mL}} = \frac{\overset{\downarrow}{DM}}{x \text{ mL}}$$

$$\frac{7\frac{1}{2} \text{ gr}}{5 \text{ mL}} = \frac{500 \text{ mg}}{x \text{ mL}}$$

Change 500 mg to gr so that the unit labels in the numerators match.

$$\frac{\overset{\downarrow}{MOH}}{5 \text{ mL}} = \frac{\overset{\downarrow}{DM}}{x \text{ mL}}$$

$$\frac{7\frac{1}{2} \text{ gr}}{5 \text{ mL}} = \frac{7\frac{1}{2} \text{ gr}}{x \text{ mL}} \leftarrow 500 \text{ mg} = 0.5 \text{ g} = 7\frac{1}{2} \text{ gr}$$

$$7\frac{1}{2}x = 7\frac{1}{2}(5)$$

$$x = 5$$

Answer. Administer to the patient 5 mL of chloral hydrate elixir (gr viiss/5 mL).

EXAMPLE 6.6

A physician prescribes potassium chloride 10 mEq diluted in 1 glass of juice qd. Potassium chloride 20 mEq per 15 mL is available in a 500 mL bottle. How many mL of potassium chloride should be dissolved in the juice?

Using Rule 6.1:

$$\frac{\overset{\downarrow}{MOH}}{15 \text{ mL}} = \frac{\overset{\downarrow}{DM}}{x \text{ mL}}$$

$$\frac{20 \text{ mEq}}{15 \text{ mL}} = \frac{10 \text{ mEq}}{x \text{ mL}}$$

$$20x = (15)(10)$$

$$x = 7\frac{1}{2} \text{ mL}$$

Answer. Dissolve $7\frac{1}{2}$ mL of potassium chloride (20 mEq/15 mL) in 1 glass of juice.

EXAMPLE 6.7

Calculate the number of mL of V-Cillin K to be administered per dose (Fig. 6–5).

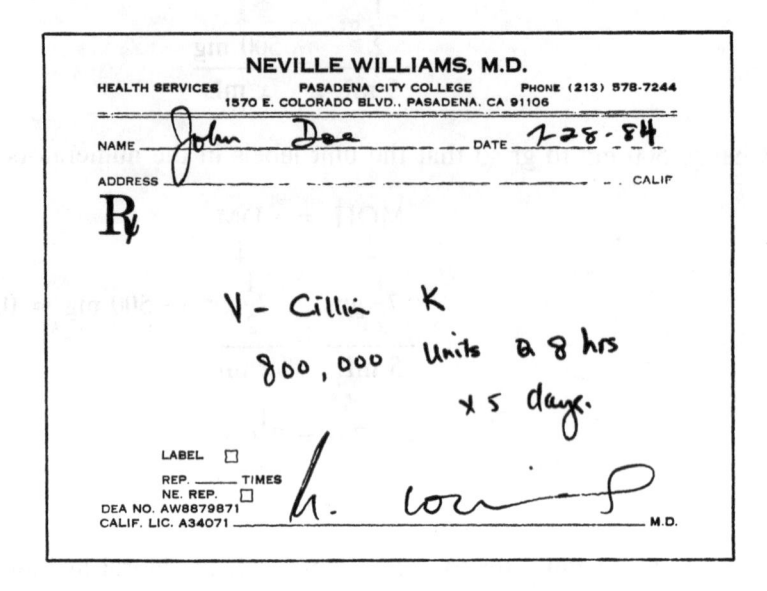

Figure 6–5. V-Cillin K prescription

> **Drug Label:** *V-Cillin K*
>
> At the time of dispensing, add 5 mL of sterile water to the dry mixture. Yields 300 000 U per 0.6 mL.

$$\begin{array}{cc} \text{MOH} & = & \text{DM} \\ \downarrow & & \downarrow \end{array}$$

$$\frac{300\,000 \text{ U}}{0.6 \text{ mL}} = \frac{800\,000 \text{ U}}{x \text{ mL}}$$

$$300\,000 x = (800\,000)(.6)$$

$$x = 1.6 \text{ mL}$$

Answer. Administer 1.6 mL of V-Cillin K (300 000 U/0.6 mL)

EXAMPLE 6.8

Calculate the correct dosage of Ilosone (Fig. 6–6).

6.2. Calculating Dosages of Oral Solutions

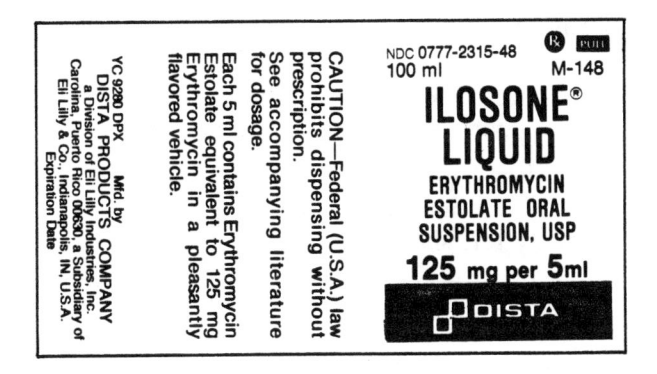

Figure 6–6. Ilosone

A physician prescribes Ilosone 0.25 g qid. How many mL should be administered?

Using Rule 6.1:

$$\text{Strength from drug label} \rightarrow \frac{\overset{MOH}{\downarrow}}{\underset{5 \text{ mL}}{125 \text{ mg}}} = \frac{\overset{DM}{\downarrow}}{\underset{x \text{ mL}}{250 \text{ mg}}}$$

$$125x = (250)(5)$$

$$x = 10 \text{ mL}$$

Answer. Administer 10 mL of Ilosone (125 mg/5 mL).

EXAMPLE 6.9

Order: Ephedrine sulfate cap ii (see Fig. 6–7). How many gr would be administered?

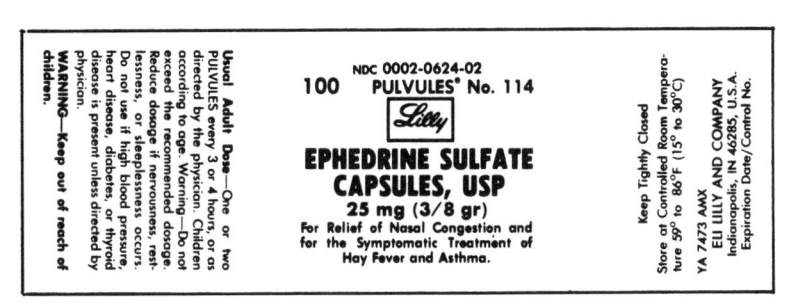

Figure 6–7. Ephedrine sulfate

Answer. Since the label states that the prescribed drug is in capsule form, simply administer 2 capsules as directed. The patient would receive gr $\frac{3}{4}$ ephedrine sulfate.

PRACTICE SET 6.2

1. A doctor prescribes 0.15 mg qd of a drug. The drug is available as 0.05 mg/mL. How many mL should be administered?

2. Drug Order: Vibramycin 75 mg po q12h.
   Available: Vibramycin 25 mg per ʒ.
   How many mL should be administered?

3. A doctor prescribes Keflex fʒ iss po q6h. Keflex oral suspension is available 125 mg/5 mL. How many mg will be administered per dose?

4. Calculate the correct dosage of Ilosone to be administered (Fig. 6–8).

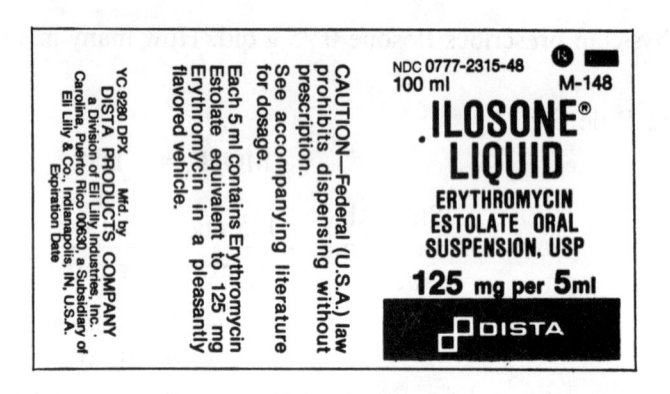

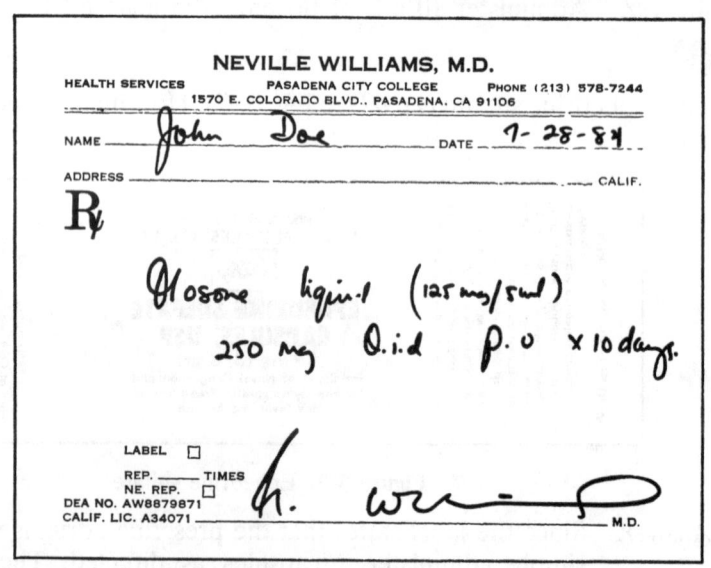

Figure 6–8. Ilosone and prescription

6.2. Calculating Dosages of Oral Solutions

5. Order: Betalin 12 Crystalline 0.3 mg total in three equally divided doses (Fig. 6-9). How many cc will you administer per dose?

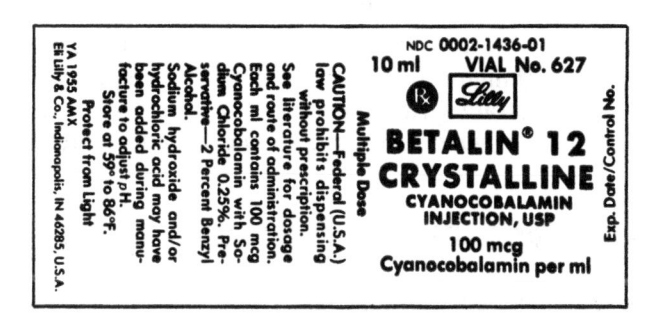

Figure 6-9. Betalin 12 Crystalline

6. Order: KCl (potassium chloride) 15 mEq po qd.
Available: KCl 20 mEq per ʒ.
How many *drams* should be administered?

7. A doctor prescribes Lasix 0.8 mL po bid c̄ meals. If Lasix is available as an oral suspension of 10 mg/mL, how many mg will be administered to the patient?

8. Chloral hydrate elixir is available 250 mg/5 mL (Fig. 6-10). How many mL should be administered to John Doe?

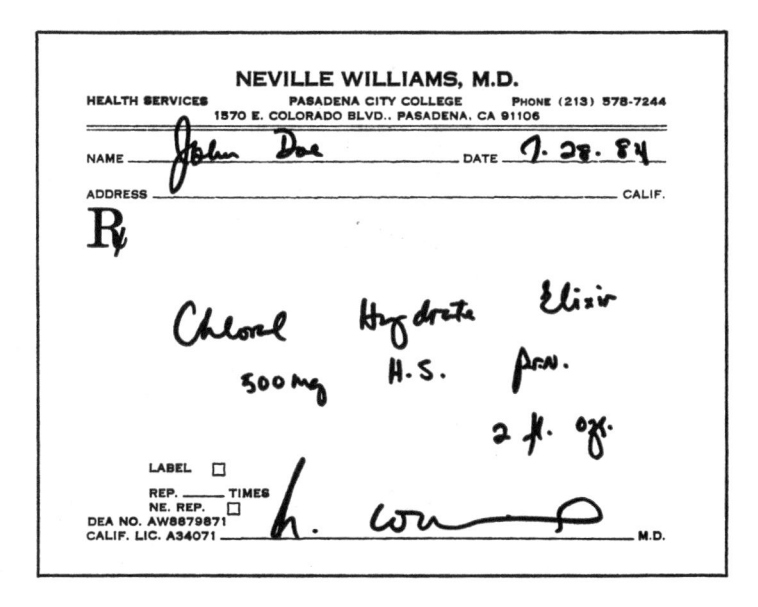

Figure 6-10. Chloral hydrate prescription

9. Order: Sulfadiazine 2 g/m² body surface for a patient with 0.8 m² body surface. Sulfadiazine in an oral suspension is available 250 mg/mL. How many mL should be administered?

10. A patient with a body surface of 0.8 m² has been ordered hydrocodone bitartrate 10 mg/m² body surface po in two equally divided doses. Hydrocodone bitartrate syrup is available in 1 mg/5 mL and 2 mg/5 mL solutions. How much of which strength should be administered per dose?

6.3 CALCULATING DOSAGES OF INJECTABLE DRUGS

When drugs cannot be administered orally, or if rapid action is desired, the drugs are given parenterally. **Parenteral** is defined as outside the alimentary canal. (The alimentary canal is the food-carrying tubular passage extending from the mouth to the anus.) Injection into the body tissue is the usual way of administering medications parenterally. These parenteral medications are absorbed directly into the bloodstream, thus enabling the body to use the drug more quickly. Another advantage of this administration route is that the drugs can be administered to unconscious or irrational patients.

There are three common types of injections: (a) subcutaneous (SC)—injections into the tissue directly under the skin; (b) intramuscular (IM)—injections into the muscle; and (c) intravenous (IV)—injections into the vein (Fig. 6–11A).

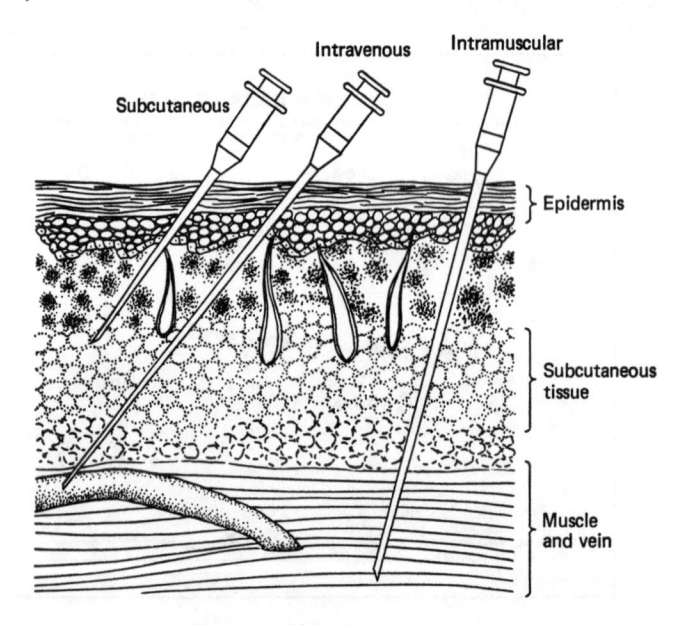

Figure 6–11A. Injection routes

6.3. Calculating Dosages of Injectable Drugs

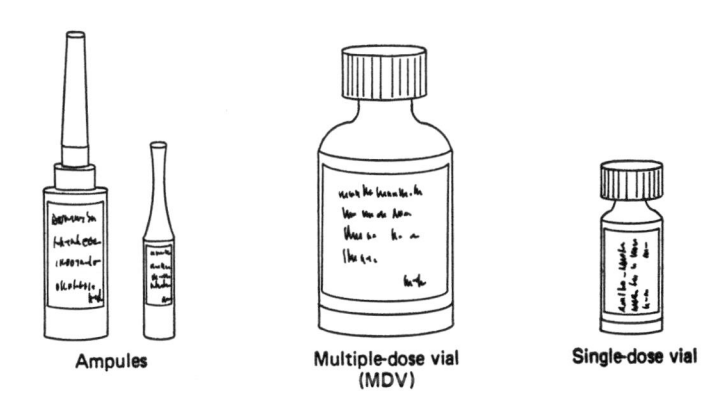

Figure 6–11B. Ampules and vials

Injectable drugs are available in both liquid and powder form. Powders must be reconstituted so that the powder is completely dissolved. Liquid drugs are usually packaged in single-dose sealed glass containers called **ampules,** or in single- or multiple-dose rubber-stoppered glass bottles called **vials.** Single-dose liquid medications may also be sealed within disposable syringes (Fig. 6–11B).

Most injectable drugs will be labeled, stating the amount of drug in the solution. It is important that you read each label carefully before you calculate parenteral dosages.

The rule for computing parenteral dosages is the same rule that was used in computing oral dosages. Since the medications will be administered using a syringe, it is first necessary that you be able to read a syringe accurately. Study the syringes shown in Figures 6–12, 6–13, and 6–14.

This syringe is calibrated in 0.1 cc units. (Fig. 6–12.)

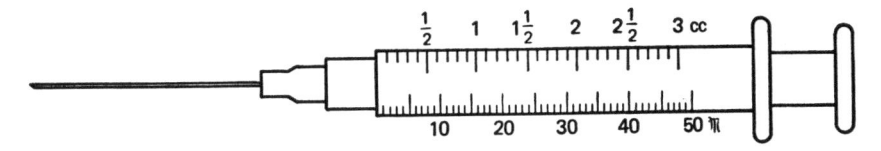

Figure 6–12. 3 cc syringe

This syringe is calibrated in 0.01 cc units. (Fig. 6–13.)

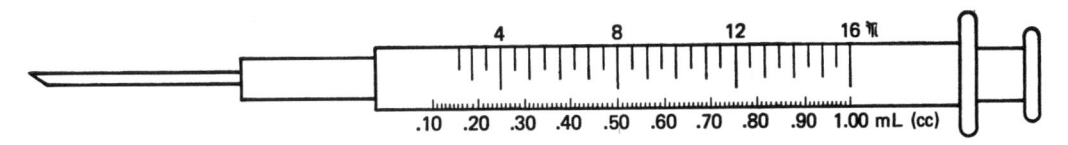

Figure 6–13. 1 cc syringe

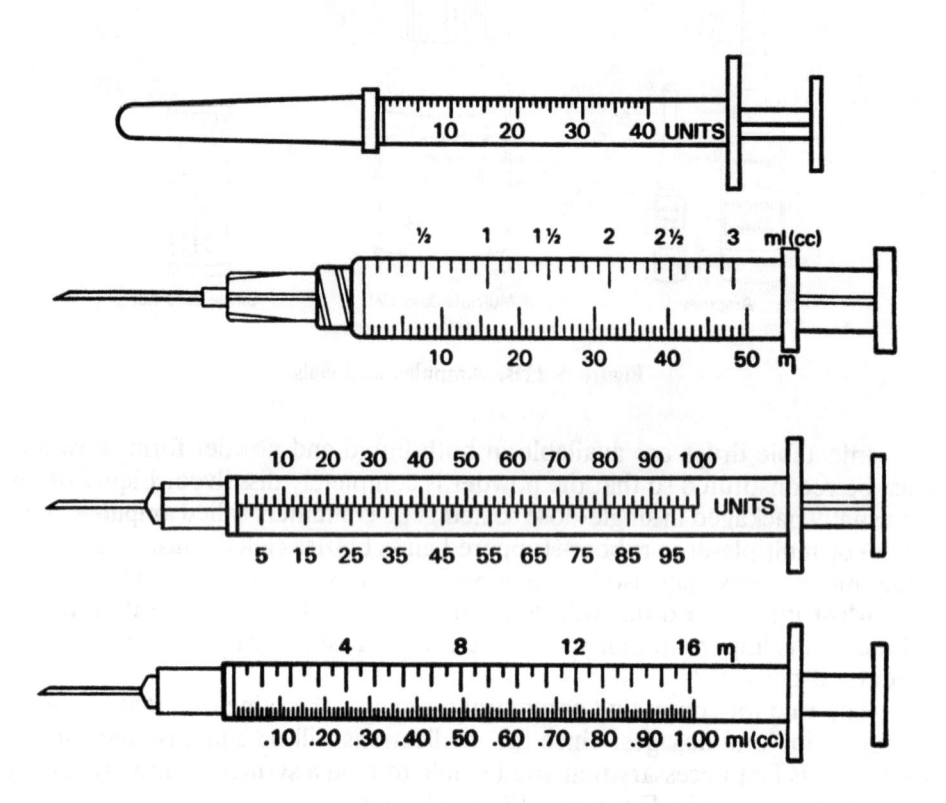

Figure 6–14. Different types of syringes

EXAMPLE 6.10

Calculate the correct dose of morphine for J. Gonzalez.

Drug Card	Drug Label
Name: J. Gonzalez Room: 16 Drug: Morphine Dose: 12 mg Route: IM Time: q4h prn	Morphine 10 mg/cc

6.3. Calculating Dosages of Injectable Drugs

$$\underset{\downarrow}{MOH} = \underset{\downarrow}{DM}$$

$$\frac{10 \text{ mg}}{1 \text{ cc}} = \frac{12 \text{ mg}}{x \text{ cc}}$$

$$10x = (12)(1)$$

$$x = 1.2 \text{ cc}$$

Administration: Draw up 1.2 cc of morphine (10 mg/cc) in a syringe and administer. The syringe shows the desired amount (Fig. 6–15).

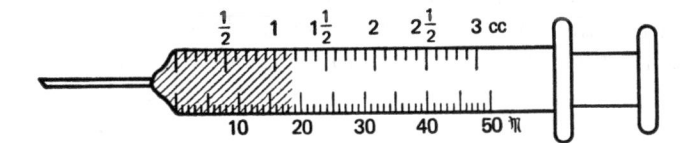

Figure 6–15. 3 cc syringe

Since this syringe is calibrated in 0.1 cc units, 1.2 cc would be two calibrations past the 1 cc mark.

EXAMPLE 6.11

A physician orders atropine 0.3 mg IM. The atropine vial reads atropine gr $\frac{1}{150}$ per mL. How many mL should be administered?

$$\underset{\downarrow}{MOH} = \underset{\downarrow}{DM}$$

$$\frac{\frac{1}{150} \text{ gr}}{1 \text{ mL}} = \frac{0.3 \text{ mg}}{x \text{ mL}}$$

Change 0.3 mg to gr and substitute this amount in the proportion:

$$\frac{1}{150} \text{ gr} \rightarrow \underset{\downarrow}{\frac{0.0067 \text{ gr}}{1 \text{ mL}}} = \underset{\downarrow}{\frac{0.005 \text{ gr}}{x \text{ ML}}} \leftarrow 0.3 \text{ mg}$$

$$0.0067x = (0.005)(1)$$

$$x = 0.75 \text{ mL}$$

Administration: Draw up 0.75 mL of atropine $\left(\frac{1}{150} \text{ gr/mL}\right)$ and administer.

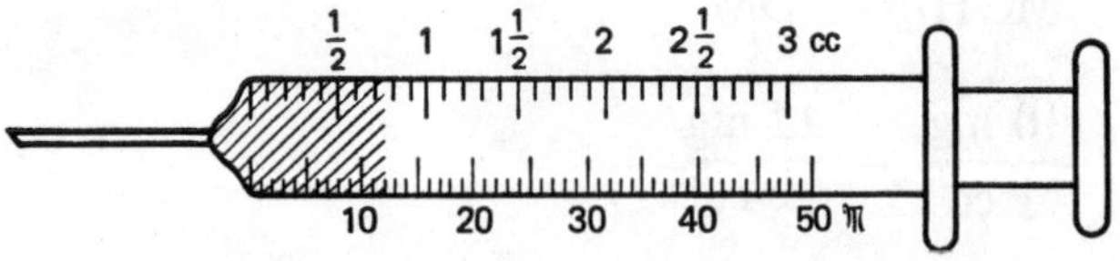

Figure 6-16. 3 cc syringe

The syringe indicates the correct dosage (Fig. 6–16).

When reconstituting parenteral drugs, it is most important that you read the directions on the label so that you know how to reconstitute the drug. The label on the vial will generally state the correct solvent to use. The usual solvents are sterile water, 0.9% sodium chloride, or bacteriostatic water. Sometimes, if a special solvent is required, the solvent is supplied along with the drug. In addition to stating the type of solvent to be used, the labels of reconstituted drugs will also state the directions for dissolving the drug. The following examples will demonstrate how parenteral drugs can be reconstituted. Reconstituted drugs should always be dated.

EXAMPLE 6.12

An order is written for Loridine 600 mg IM. The drug label reads, "Loridine equivalent to 1 gr. Add 2.5 mL of sterile water for injection. Yields 3.3 mL reconstituted solution containing 300 mg/mL."

Strength after the reconstitution ⟶

$$\text{MOH} = \text{DM}$$
$$\frac{300 \text{ mg}}{1 \text{ mL}} = \frac{600 \text{ mg}}{x \text{ mL}}$$
$$300x = (600)(1)$$
$$x = 2 \text{ mL}$$

Administration: Inject 2.5 mL of sterile water into the 1 g vial of Loridine and shake well to dissolve; withdraw 2 mL and administer.

EXAMPLE 6.13

A 2 g vial of ampicillin is available. The reconstitution directions read, "Add 6.8 cc of sterile water for injection to contents of vial. Resulting solution has strength of 0.25 g/cc." A physician orders 300 mg IM, q6h for a patient. Write the administration for the patient.

Strength after the reconstitution ⟶

$$\text{MOH} = \text{DM}$$
$$\frac{0.25 \text{ g}}{1 \text{ cc}} = \frac{0.3 \text{ g}}{x \text{ cc}} \leftarrow 300 \text{ mg}$$
$$0.25x = (0.3)(1)$$
$$x = 1.2 \text{ cc}$$

6.3. Calculating Dosages of Injectable Drugs

Administration: Inject 6.8 cc of sterile water into the 2 g vial of ampicillin and shake well to dissolve; withdraw 1.2 cc and administer.

Insulin is a drug that must be administered parenterally because it is destroyed in the gastrointestinal tract. It is a highly sensitive drug and thus mandates exact dosages.

Insulin is measured in units and comes in various strengths, such as U-40 (40 units/mL), U-80 (80 units/mL), U-100 (100 units/mL), or U-500 (500 units/mL). Both U-40 and U-80 have been phased out and are no longer used. In administering U-100 insulin, a U-100 syringe should be used. If a U-100 syringe is not available, then a tuberculin or hypodermic syringe can be used. You should be able to administer insulin using either the U-100 or the tuberculin syringe. Study the U-100 syringe in Figure 6–17.

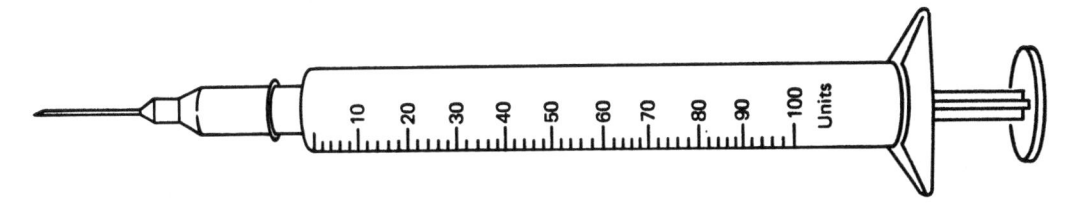

Figure 6–17. U-100 insulin syringe

This syringe can deliver 1 mL containing 100 units of insulin. Each calibration is 2 units.

EXAMPLE 6.14

Order: 50 units of U-100 regular insulin. Administer in a U-100 syringe. Shade in the correct dosage on the syringe.

Answer. Since a U-100 syringe is available, use it to administer the U-100 insulin. It is calibrated for U-100 insulin (Fig. 6–18).

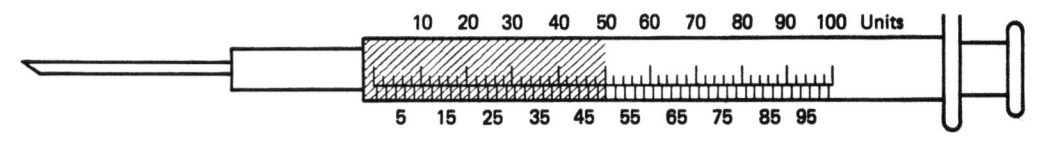

Figure 6–18. U-100 syringe

Shade in 50 units on the U-100 syringe.

Whenever a U-100 syringe is not available for administering U-100 insulin, a tuberculin or a hypodermic syringe is used.

144 6. Calculations for Oral and Parenteral Dosages

EXAMPLE 6.15

Order: 45 units of U-100 regular insulin. Administer using a 1 cc tuberculin syringe. Shade in the correct dosage.

The strength (U-100) of the insulin is equivalent to the medication on hand. U-100 means 100 units insulin per mL. The desired medication is 45 units. Find the number of cc that contains 45 units (Fig. 6–19).

$$\text{MOH} = \text{DM}$$

Strength of U-100 insulin $\longrightarrow$

$$\frac{100 \text{ U}}{1 \text{ cc}} = \frac{45 \text{ U}}{x \text{ cc}}$$

$$100x = (45)(1)$$

$$x = 0.45 \text{ cc}$$

Answer. Shade in 0.45 cc on the syringe.

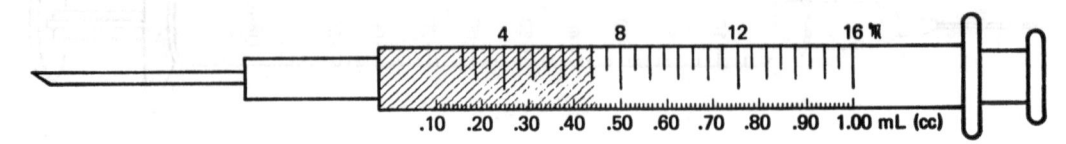

Figure 6–19. Tuberculin syringe

EXAMPLE 6.16

Order: 410 units of U-500 insulin. Administer using a 1 cc syringe. Shade in the correct dosage on the syringe (Fig. 6–20).

$$\text{MOH} = \text{DM}$$

Strength of U-500 insulin $\longrightarrow$

$$\frac{500 \text{ U}}{1 \text{ cc}} = \frac{410 \text{ U}}{x \text{ cc}}$$

$$500x = (410)(1)$$

$$x = 0.82 \text{ cc}$$

Answer. Shade in 0.82 cc on the syringe.

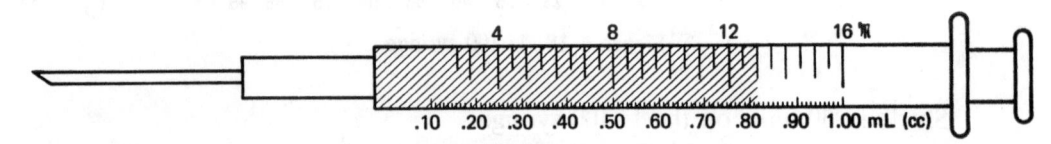

Figure 6–20. 1 cc syringe

Heparin and penicillin are two other drugs that are measured in units.

6.3. Calculating Dosages of Injectable Drugs

EXAMPLE 6.17

An order is for heparin 15 000 units SC. The medication on hand is 20 000 U/mL. Shade in the syringe to indicate the amount of heparin to be administered (Fig. 6–21).

$$\text{MOH} = \text{DM}$$

$$\frac{20\ 000\ \text{U}}{1\ \text{mL}} = \frac{15\ 000\ \text{U}}{x\ \text{mL}}$$

$$20\ 000x = (15\ 000)(1)$$

$$x = 0.75\ \text{mL}$$

Answer. Shade in 0.75 cc on the syringe.

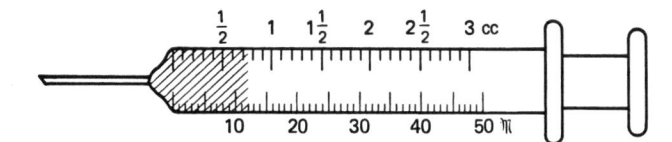

Figure 6–21. 3 cc syringe

EXAMPLE 6.18

Order: 500 000 U penicillin from a vial labeled 5 000 000 U/10 mL. Inject 8 mL of sterile water to yield 10 mL solution. How many mL should be administered? Write the administration for this drug.

$$\text{MOH} = \text{DM}$$

Reconstituted strength → $\dfrac{5\ 000\ 000\ \text{U}}{10\ \text{mL}} = \dfrac{500\ 000\ \text{U}}{x\ \text{mL}}$

$$5\ 000\ 000x = (500\ 000)(10)$$

$$x = 1\ \text{mL}$$

Administration: Inject 8 mL of sterile water into the 5 000 000 U vial of penicillin and shake well to dissolve; withdraw 1 mL and administer.

PRACTICE SET 6.3

1. Order: Staphcillin 800 mg IM.
   Medication on hand: Staphcillin 1 g. Add 1.8 mL of sterile water to yield 500 mg/mL.
   How many mL will you administer? Write the administration.

146   6. Calculations for Oral and Parenteral Dosages

2. Order: 20 000 U heparin SC abdominally q6h.
   Available: 10 mL vial heparin 40 000 U/mL.
   How many mL should be administered per dose?

3. An order of morphine sulfate is for 10 mg IM. The drug label reads morphine sulfate gr $\frac{1}{4}$/mL. Indicate how many mL should be administered by shading in the syringe in Figure 6–22.

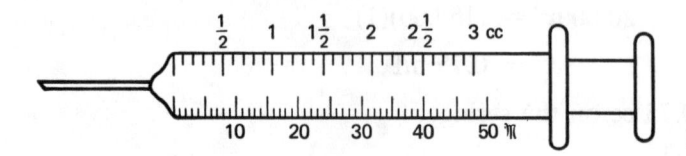

Figure 6–22. 3 cc syringe

4. Drug Order: Penicillin G potassium 125 000 U q6h.
   Form available: 1 000 000 U vial (powder).
   If the powder is dissolved in 3.6 mL of sterile water, there will be 250 000 U/mL. How many mL should be given per dose?

5. Order: Sodium Luminal 65 mg IM.
   Medication on hand: Sodium Luminal 130 mg/2 cc.
   How many cc should be administered? Shade in the answer (Fig. 6–23).

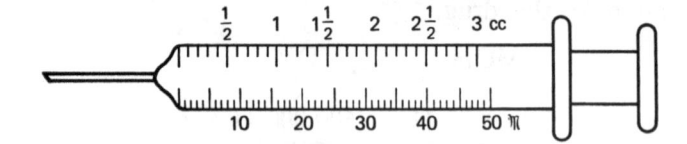

Figure 6–23. 3 cc syringe

6. A physician orders Demerol 30 mg IM. Demerol 0.05 g/mL is available. How many mL are needed?

7. Drug Order: Penicillin G potassium 600 000 U q6h.
   Form available: Pencillin G potassium 1 000 000 U vial of powder. If powder is dissolved in 3.8 mL of sterile water, there will be 200 000 U/mL. How many mL should be administered?

8. A doctor prescribes 60 units of U-100 isophane insulin for a patient. A tuberculin syringe is available. How many mL should be administered? Shade in the answer. (Fig. 6–24).

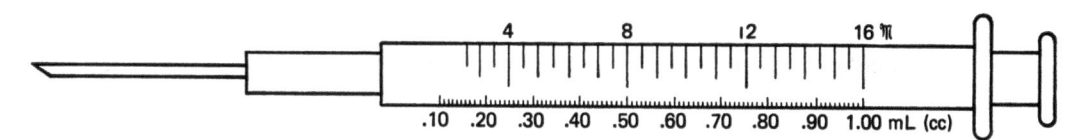

Figure 6-24. 1 cc syringe

9. A diabetic patient is to receive 70 units of U-100 NPH Iletin. Shade in the U-100 syringe to designate the correct dosage. (Fig. 6-25).

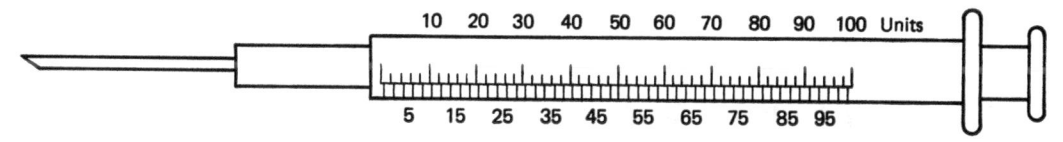

Figure 6-25. U-100 syringe

10. A doctor prescribes 250 U of U-500 insulin for a patient requiring an immediate high dosage of insulin. Indicate on the syringe how many mL should be administered (Fig. 6-26).

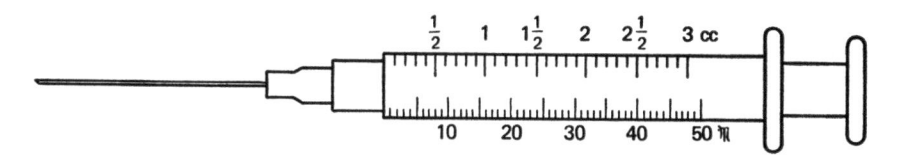

Figure 6-26. 3 cc syringe

6.4 CHAPTER 6 REVIEW PROBLEMS

1. Order: 45 units of U-100 regular insulin. Administer in 1 cc syringe. Shade in the correct dosage (Fig 6-27).

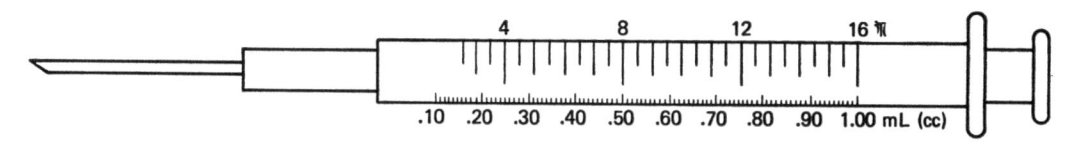

Figure 6-27. 1 cc syringe

2. Order: Vitamin A 150 units in three equally divided doses. Forms available: Vitamin A 50 unit/tab and 150 unit/tab. How many tabs should be administered per dose?

3. Calculate the correct dosage of Crysticillin (Fig. 6–28).

```
NEVILLE WILLIAMS, M.D.
HEALTH SERVICES   PASADENA CITY COLLEGE   PHONE (213) 578-7244
       1570 E. COLORADO BLVD., PASADENA, CA 91106

NAME  John Doe              DATE  7-28-84
ADDRESS _____ CALIF.

Rx
    Crysticillin Suspension
    450,000 Units I.m daily
                       x 7 days.

LABEL ☐
REP. ____ TIMES
NE. REP. ☐                  M. Corwin, M.D.
DEA NO. AW8879871
CALIF. LIC. A34071
```

Drug Label

Crysticillin
300 000 U/cc

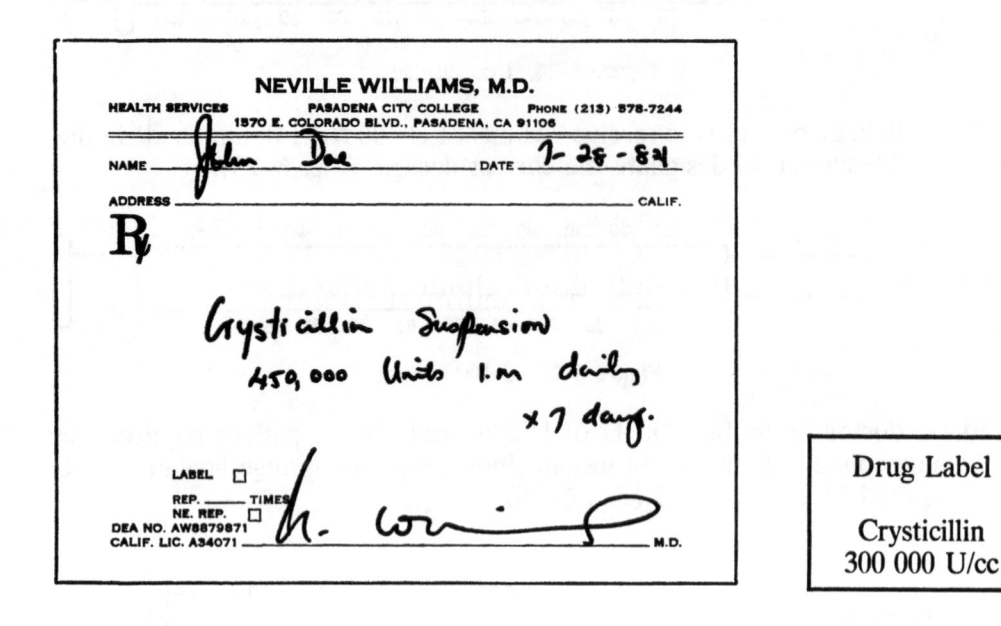

Figure 6–28. Crysticillin prescription

4. Order: 250 units of U-500 insulin. Administer using a 1 cc syringe. Shade in the correct dosage (Fig. 6–29).

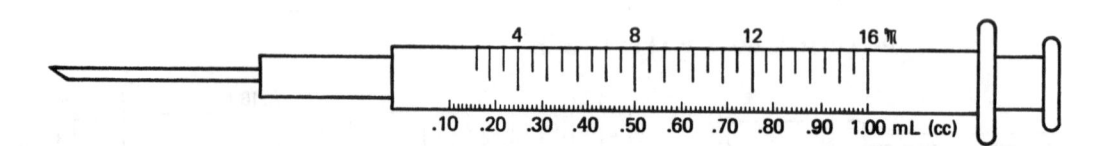

Figure 6–29. 1 cc syringe

5. A doctor orders Klorvess 30 mEq diluted in juice qd. The pharmacy has available Klorvess 20 mEq per 15 mL. How many mL will be administered to the patient?

6.4. Chapter 6 Review Problems   149

6. Calculate the correct number of tablets of V-Cillin K to be ordered from the pharmacy for this prescription (Fig. 6–30) for five days.

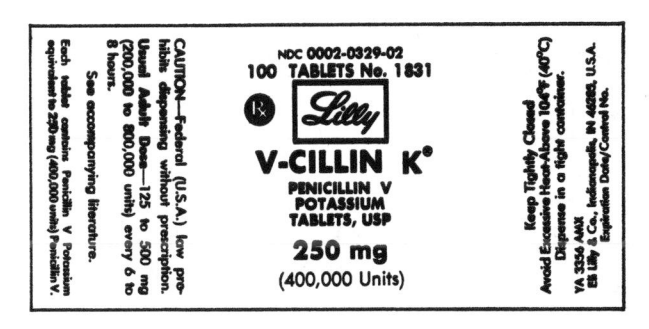

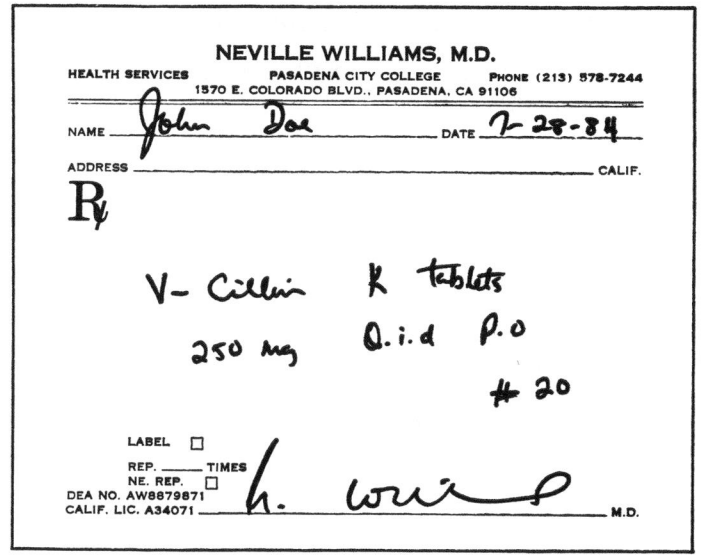

Figure 6–30. V-Cillin K and prescription

7. Order: 75 units of U-100 regular insulin. Shade in the correct setting on the syringe (Fig. 6–31).

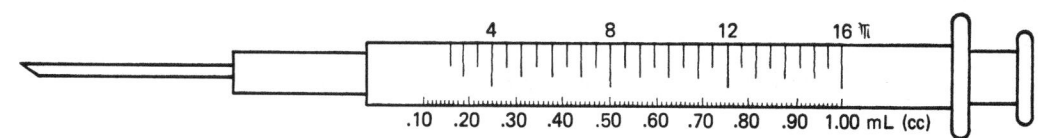

Figure 6–31. 1 cc syringe

8. A physician has ordered penicillin G 600 000 U IM. The drug label reads 400 000 U/mL. Shade the syringe to indicate how many mL would be administered (Fig. 6–32).

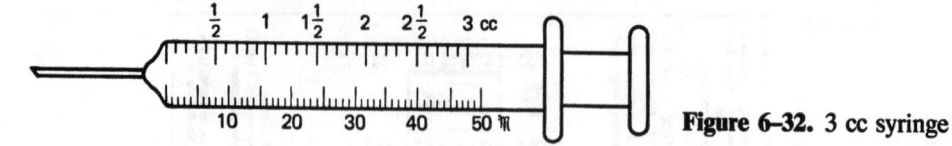

Figure 6–32. 3 cc syringe

9. Order: Bleomycin 15 units/m² body surface.
Available: Bleomycin 10 units/mL. The patient has 1.8 m² body surface. How many mL should be administered?

10. A doctor prescribes Thyroid USP gr iss tablets. How many Thyroid USP tablets gr ss should be administered?

11. Calculate the correct dose of morphine sulfate. The drug label reads morphine sulfate 10 mg/mL (Fig. 6–33).

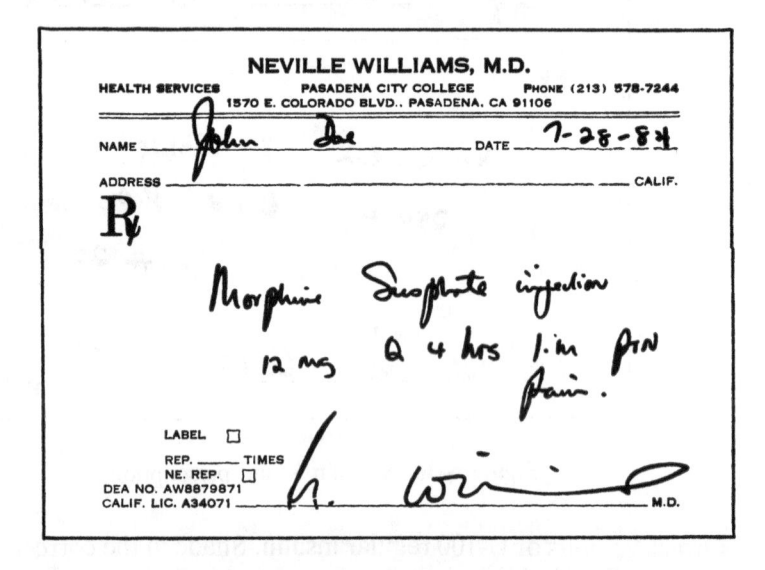

Figure 6–33. Morphine sulfate prescription

12. An order calls for 60 mg of atropine sulfate from a 2 cc ampule labeled 0.3 g/2 cc. How many cc should be administered?

13. Drug order: 300 mg sodium bicarbonate.
Medication on hand: Sodium bicarbonate gr v/5 mL.
How many mL should be administered?

6.4. Chapter 6 Review Problems

14. Administer 500 mg of sodium ampicillin from a vial labeled "1 g, inject 2.4 mL sterile water to yield 2.5 mL of solution." Write the administration.

15. Administer 60 units of U-100 regular insulin. Shade in the syringe to indicate the correct answer (Fig. 6–34).

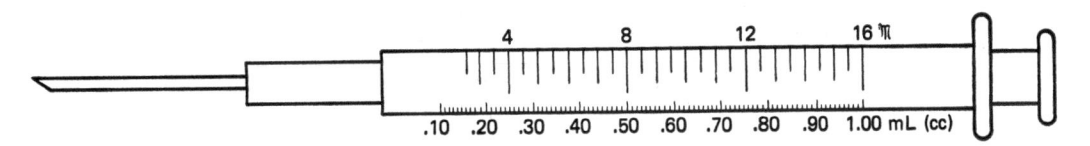

Figure 6–34. 1 cc syringe

16. Order: 65 000 units penicillin G potassium per kg body mass per day in two equally divided doses.
    Medication on hand: Pencillin G potassium 2 000 000 U/mL.
    How many mL/dose should be administered to a 105.6-lb patient? Shade in the correct answer on the syringe (Fig. 6–35).

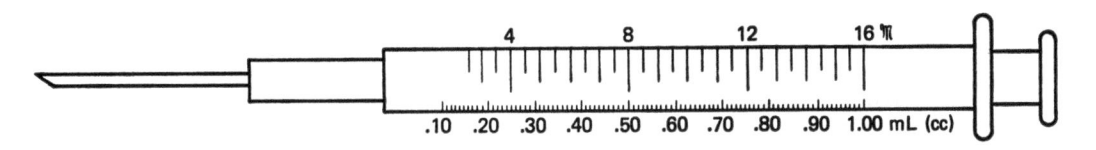

Figure 6–35. 1 cc syringe

17. Order: Bleomycin 12 units/m^2 body surface.
    Medication on hand: 10 units/mL.
    How many mL should be administered to a patient with 1.5 m^2 body surface?

18. | Drug Label | | Drug order: 70 mg IM Droiban IM |
    | Drolban |
    | 50 mg/mL |

    How many mL should be administered per dose?

19. Drug order: 150 mg Benadryl.
    Available: Benadryl 50 mg capsules.
    How many capsules should be administered?

152   6. Calculations for Oral and Parenteral Dosages

20. Drug order: 130 mg Darvon (Fig. 6–36).
How many capsules should be administered?

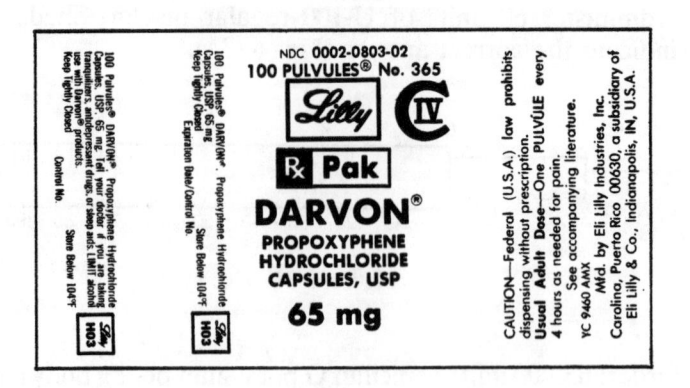

Figure 6–36. Darvon

21. Order: Nembutal gr iii po hs.
Available: Nembutal capsules gr $\frac{3}{4}$.
How many Nembutal capsules should be administered?

22. Order: Aspirin gr xv po qid.
Available: Aspirin 300 mg tablets.
How many tablets should be administered?

23. Order: Stilbestrol 0.5 mg qd (Fig. 6–37).
How many tabs should be administered?

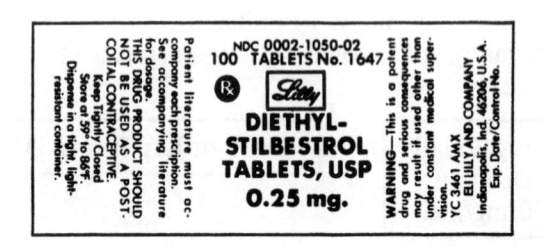

Figure 6–37. Stilbestrol

24. Order: 37 units of U-100 regular insulin. Administer in a 1 cc syringe. Shade in the syringe to indicate the correct dosage (Fig. 6–38).

6.4. Chapter 6 Review Problems

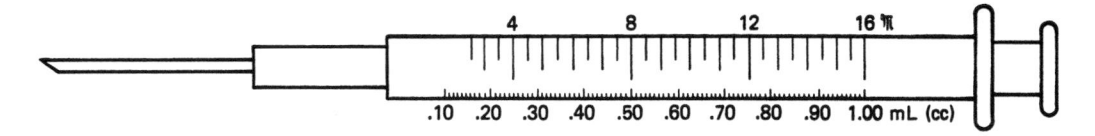

Figure 6-38. 1 cc syringe

25. Order: Meperidine hydrochloride 45 mg IM q4h.
    Available: Meperidine hydrochloride ampule 25 mg/0.5 mL.
    Shade in the syringe to indicate the correct dosage (Fig. 6-39).

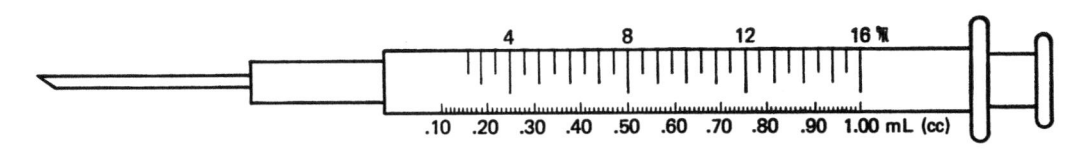

Figure 6-39. 1 cc syringe

26. Aqueous penicillin G 500 000 U IM q6h is prescribed for a patient. The vial reads:

    > Pencillin G. potassium injection
    > 1 000 000 U/vial

    Reconstitution: Add 4.6 mL of normal saline to contents of vial. Resultant solution is 200 000 U/mL. How many mL should be administered to the patient?

27. A doctor prescribes 50 000 units of heparin for a patient to prevent the possibility of thromboemboli formation. It is to be administered SC two hours before surgery, then q8h. Heparin 40 000 U/mL is available. How many mL should be administered to the patient before surgery?

28. Order: Demerol 50 mg IM q4h prn.
    Available: Demerol vial 100 mg/2 mL.
    How many mL should be administered?

29. Loridine 600 mg IM q12h is ordered for a patient. Loridine must be reconstituted according to the following directions: Add 2.5 mL of sterile water for injection. The resultant solution is 300 mg/mL. Write the administration for this drug.

154   6. Calculations for Oral and Parenteral Dosages

30. Calculate the correct dose of atropine sulfate for the patient (Fig. 6–40).

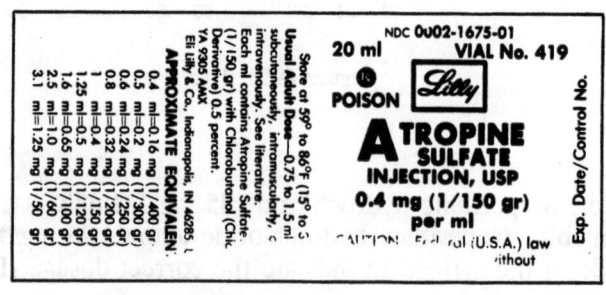

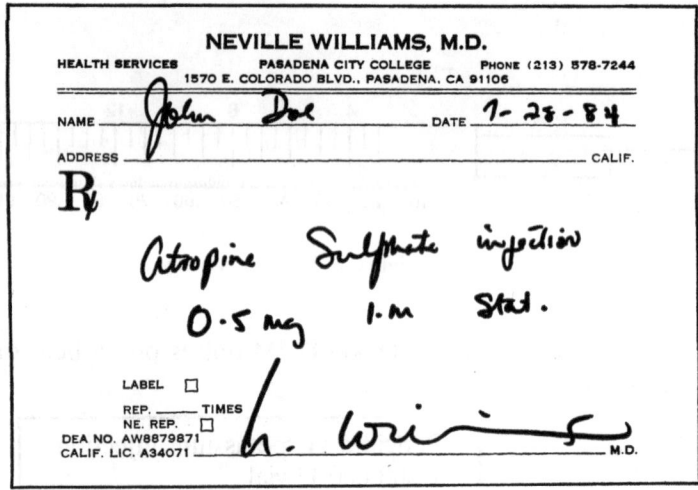

Figure 6–40. Atropine sulfate and prescription

31.
Drug Label
Crysticillin
300 000 U/cc

Order: Crysticillin 450 000 U IM bid.
How many cc should be administered?

32. Order: Digoxin 100 mcg IM qid.
Available: Digoxin 0.5 mg/2 mL.
How many mL should be administered?

33. Order: Neotrizine 2000 mg stat, then 1000 mg q6h (Fig. 6–41). How many tablets should be administered stat? How many tablets should be administered q6h?

6.4. Chapter 6 Review Problems

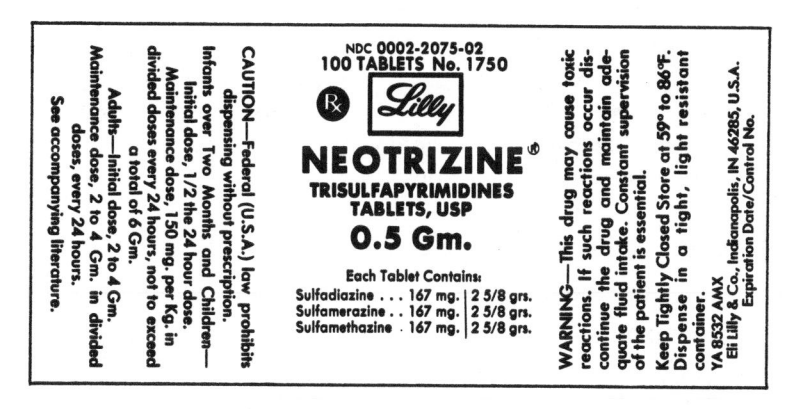

Figure 6–41. Neotrizine

34. Order: 48 000 U heparin.
    Available: 5 mL vial of heparin 20 000 U/mL.
    Shade in the syringe to show the correct dosage (Fig. 6–42).

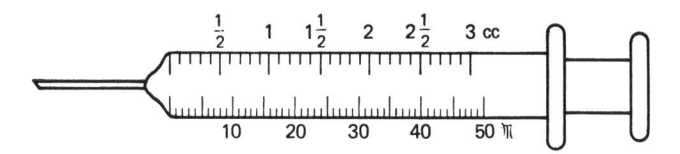

    Figure 6–42. 3 cc syringe

35. Order: 375 units of U-500 insulin.
    Administer using a 1 cc syringe. Shade in the syringe to show the correct dosage (Fig. 6–43).

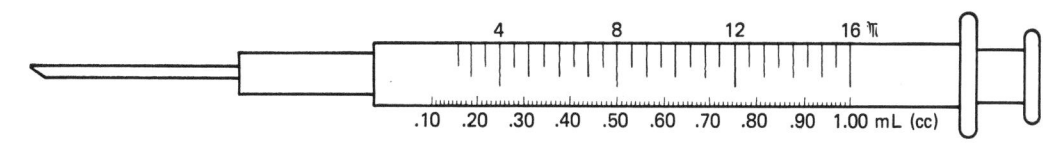

    Figure 6–43. 1 cc syringe

36. A diabetic is to receive 55 units of U-100 insulin. You have only a tuberculin syringe available. How many cc should you administer using this syringe? Shade in the correct amount in the syringe (Fig. 6–44).

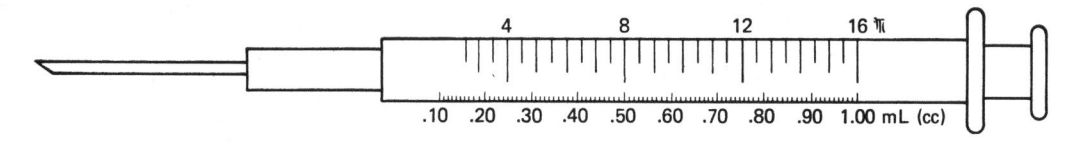

    Figure 6–44. 1 cc syringe

37. Order: Ampicillin 50 mg IM q6h.
Available: A 125 mg vial of ampicillin sodium injection. Reconstitution: Add 1.2 mL of sterile water for injection to contents of vial. The resulting solution strength is 125 mg/mL.
How many mL should be administered?

38. Order: Dilaudid gr $\frac{1}{15}$ SC q3h.
Available: Dilaudid 3 mg/mL.
How many ♏ should be administered?

39. Order: KCl 20 mEq po bid.
Available: Liquid KCl 40 mEq/30 mL.
How many mL should be administered?

6.5 CHAPTER 6 SELF TEST

6.2 **1.** Order: Neo-Betalin Crystalline 0.5 cc IM (Fig. 6–45). How many mg should be administered?

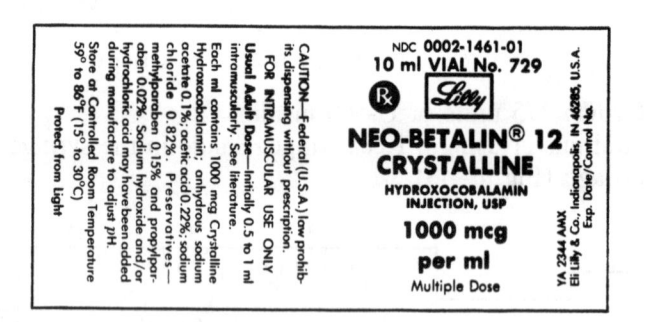

Figure 6–45. Neo-Betalin Crystalline

6.3 **2.** A physician has ordered pencillin G sodium 600 000 U IM. The drug label reads 400 000 U/mL. Shade the syringe to indicate how many mL should be administered (Fig. 6–46).

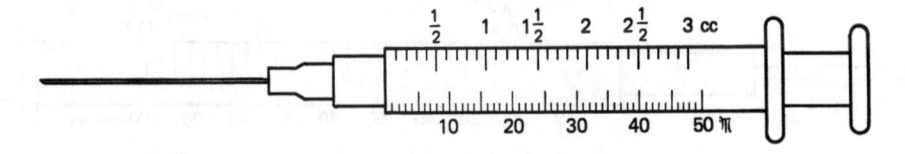

Figure 6–46. 3 cc syringe

6.5. Chapter 6 Self Test

6.1 **3.** Order: Seconal Sodium gr iii (Fig. 6–47). How many tabs should be administered per dose?

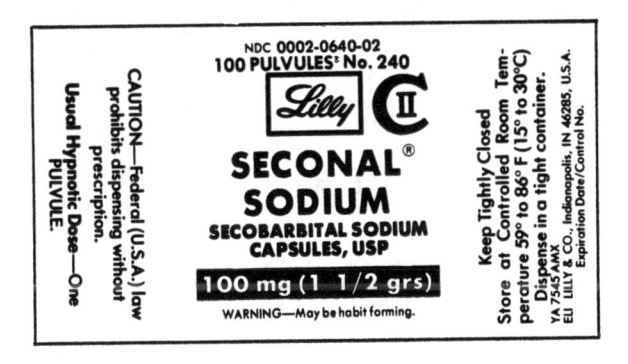

Figure 6–47. Seconal Sodium

6.3 **4.** Order: 65 units of U-100 regular insulin in a 100-unit syringe. Shade in the correct syringe setting for the administration (Fig. 6–48).

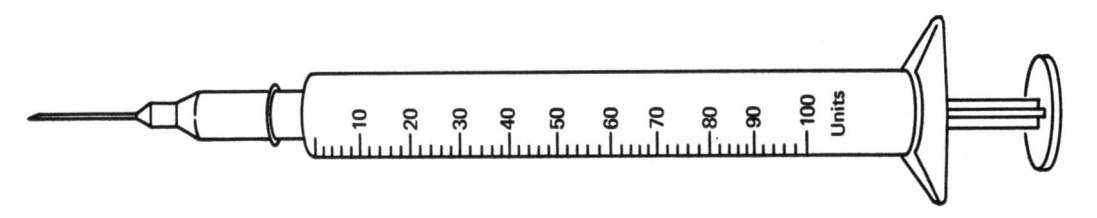

Figure 6–48. U-100 syringe

6.1 **5.** Order: Crystodigin gr $\frac{1}{600}$ po qd.

Available: Crystodigin scored tabs gr $\frac{1}{300}$.

How many tabs should be administered per dose? _____

6.2 **6.** Order: Loridine gr iiss IM (Fig. 6–49).
Administration: _____

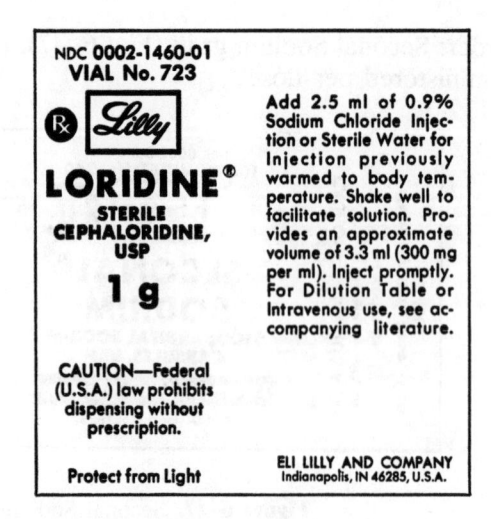

158   6. Calculations for Oral and Parenteral Dosages

```
NDC 0002-1460-01
VIAL No. 723

℞  Lilly

LORIDINE®
   STERILE
CEPHALORIDINE,
     USP

     1 g

Add 2.5 ml of 0.9%
Sodium Chloride Injec-
tion or Sterile Water for
Injection previously
warmed to body tem-
perature. Shake well to
facilitate solution. Pro-
vides an approximate
volume of 3.3 ml (300 mg
per ml). Inject promptly.
For Dilution Table or
Intravenous use, see ac-
companying literature.

CAUTION—Federal
(U.S.A.) law prohibits
dispensing without
prescription.

Protect from Light         ELI LILLY AND COMPANY
                           Indianapolis, IN 46285, U.S.A.
```

Figure 6–49. Loridine

6.2 **7.** Order: Heparin 4000 U SC q6h.
     Available: Heparin 40 000 U/mL.
     How many mL should be administered per dose?
     _____

6.2 **8.** Administer 75 mg Vistaril po tid. Vistaril oral suspension is available 30 mg/tsp. How many tsp should be administered per dose?
     _____

6.3 **9.** Order: 27 units of U-100 regular insulin. Shade in the correct setting on the syringe (Fig. 6–50).

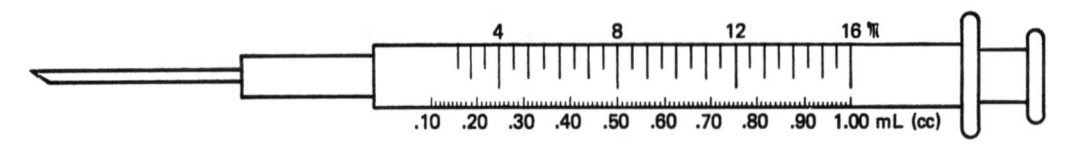

Figure 6–50. 1 cc syringe

6.1 **10.** Order: Gantrisin 2 g po tid.
      Available: Gantrisin gr viiss tablets.
      How many tabs should be administered per dose?
      _____

6.2 **11.** A doctor prescribes V-Cillin K 500 000 U po q6h. If 200 000 U per ʒ is available, how many ʒ should be administered per dose?
      _____

6.5. Chapter 6 Self Test   159

6.2 **12.** Order: KCl 25 mEq po bid.
Available: KCl 20 mEq/30 mL.
How many mL should be administered per dose? _____

6.2 **13.** Order: Decadron-LA 4 mg IM
Available: Decadron-LA 8 mg/mL (Fig. 6–51)
How many cc should be administered? _____

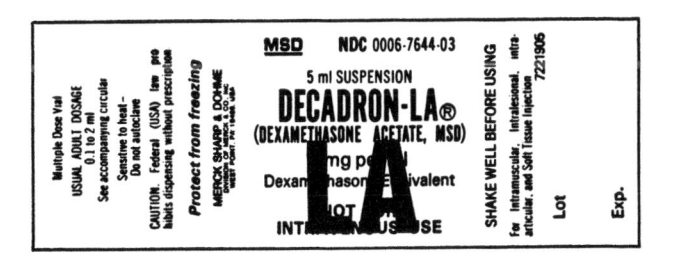

Figure 6–51. Decadron-LA

6.3 **14.** A doctor has prescribed 350 mg Oxacillin IM q4h. The label for a 500 mg vial of Oxacillin reads, "Add 2.7 cc of sterile water for injection to contents of vial. The resultant strength of solution is 250 mg/1.5 cc." Shade in the syringe to show the correct amount per dose (Fig. 6–52).

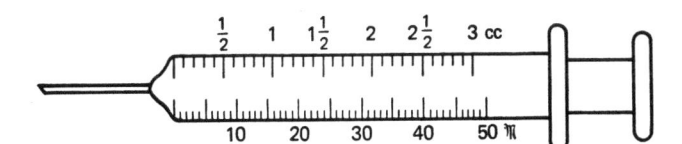

Figure 6–52. 3 cc syringe

6.1 **15.** Order: 40 000 U penicillin G potassium/kg body mass administered daily po in three equally divided doses. Pencillin G potassium is available as 100 000 U/tab, 250 000 U/tab, and 500 000 U/tab. Which kind and how many tabs should be administered to an $82\frac{1}{2}$-lb patient per dose? _____

SUMMARY OF CHAPTER 6 RULES

RULE 6.1 Rule for Calculating Tablet and Capsule Dosage

Step 1. Write the medication on hand (MOH) as a ratio.

Step 2. Write the desired medication (DM) as a ratio.

Step 3. Set the two ratios equal to each other and solve for x.

7
Calculations for Intravenous Fluids

OBJECTIVES

After studying this chapter you should be able to

1. calculate the rate of flow for IV fluids;
2. calculate the running time for IV fluids;
3. solve problems involving piggyback IVs.

INTRODUCTION

Intravenous (IV) administration delivers drugs by a drop method over an extended period of time directly into the bloodstream. The drugs are injected into the patient's circulatory system via selected veins. Once the fluids are injected into the veins, they are carried throughout the body in a matter of minutes, allowing for fast absorption by the body.

The most common way that IV fluids are administered to a patient is via an IV administration set. Administration sets are calibrated in drops per mL. You should check each administration set before using it, since different manufacturers produce IV sets that yield a varying number of drops per mL. For example, the Baxter set yields 10 gtt/mL, the Culter set yields 20 gtt/mL and the microdropper yields 60 gtt/mL. The drop factor varies because of the size of the opening of the particular drip chamber.

Four factors must be considered in administering IV fluids:
1. The number of *milliliters* to be administered
2. The calibration of the administration set in *gtt/mL*
3. The rate of flow calculated in *gtt/min*
4. The running time calculated in *minutes*

7.1 CALCULATING THE RATE OF FLOW

When an IV order is written, the physician orders a certain amount of fluid to be administered over a fixed period of time. You should be able to calculate the rate of flow.

> **RULE 7.1 Rule for Calculating the Rate of Flow for IV Fluids**
>
> $$\text{Rate of flow} = \frac{(\text{Amount of fluid})(\text{Administration set calibration})}{\text{Running time}}$$
>
> $$\frac{x}{1} = \frac{(\text{mL})(\text{gtt/mL})}{\text{min}}$$

When the formula is used, all the unit labels cancel except gtt/min, which is the correct unit label for the rate of flow.

$$\frac{x}{1} = \frac{(\text{mL})\left(\frac{\text{gtt}}{\text{mL}}\right)}{\text{min}}$$

$$\frac{x}{1} = \frac{\left(\frac{\cancel{\text{mL}}}{1}\right)\left(\frac{\text{gtt}}{\cancel{\text{mL}}}\right)}{\text{min}}$$

$$x = \frac{\text{gtt}}{\text{min}}$$

EXAMPLE 7.1

A physician orders 1500 mL of isotonic saline solution to run over a 24-hour period. What is the rate of flow if the administration set reads 20 gtt/mL?

Total amount = 1500 mL
Administration set = 20 gtt/mL
Running time = 24 hr = 24 hr × 60 min/hr = 1440 min

7.1. Calculating the Rate of Flow

By substitution in Rule 7.1:

$$\frac{x}{1} = \frac{(1500 \text{ mL})(20 \text{ gtt/mL})}{1440 \text{ min}}$$

$$1440\, x = (1500)(20)$$

$$x = 20.83$$

Answer. Rate of flow = 20.83 gtt/min or 21 gtt/min (Round off the rate of flow to the nearest whole number.)

EXAMPLE 7.2

Order: 1 L 5% dextrose IV over 15 hr.
Administration set: 15 gtt/mL.

Total amount = 1 L = 1000 mL
Administration set = 15 gtt/mL
Running time = 15 hr = 900 min

Using Rule 7.1:

$$\frac{x}{1} = \frac{(1000 \text{ mL})(15 \text{ gtt/mL})}{900 \text{ min}}$$

$$900\, x = (1000)(15)$$

$$x = 16.66$$

Answer. Rate of flow = 16.66 or 17 gtt/min

EXAMPLE 7.3

Order: 1 L D5W (dextrose 5% in water) IV over 480 min.
Administration set: 10 gtt/mL.

Total amount = 1 L = 1000 mL
Administration set = 10 gtt/mL
Running time = 480 min

Using Rule 7.1:

$$\frac{x}{1} = \frac{(1000 \text{ mL})(10 \text{ gtt/mL})}{480 \text{ min}}$$

$$480\, x = (1000)(10)$$

$$x = 20.8$$

Answer. Rate of flow = 20.8 gt/min or 21 gtt/min

For adults, the flow rate of IV fluids is calculated in gtt/min. For infants and children, however, the flow rate is calculated in microdrops per minute. 60 **microdrops** equal 1 mL. The 60 gtt/mL set is called the microdropper administration set. Usually, a counting device is attached on such an administration set so that a dial can be used to set the desired rate of flow.

EXAMPLE 7.4

An order is for 1000 mL of $\frac{1}{6}$ molar sodium lactate IV to run 250 mL/hr. If a microdropper administration set is used, how many microdrops per min should the IV drip?

Total amount = 1000 mL
Administration set = 60 gtt/mL
Running time = ?

To calculate the number of hours, divide the total amount by the number of mL/hr.

$$\text{Total number of hr} = \frac{1000 \text{ mL}}{250 \text{ mL/hr}} = 4 \text{ hr} = 240 \text{ min}$$

Using Rule 7.1:

$$\frac{x}{1} = \frac{(1000 \text{ mL})(60 \text{ gtt/mL})}{240 \text{ min}}$$

$$240 x = (1000)(60)$$

$$x = 250$$

Answer. Rate of flow = 250 gtt/min

Sometimes a doctor will prescribe a continuous infusion of a given concentrated solution based on med/min or med/kg/min.

EXAMPLE 7.5

A patient is to receive 2 mg/min of an IV medication. On hand is an IV bottle labeled 600 mg/200 mL. Find the rate of flow if a microdropper administration set is used.

Step 1. Calculate the number of minutes the IV should flow.

$$\frac{2 \text{ mg}}{1 \text{ min}} = \frac{600 \text{ mg}}{x \text{ min}}$$

$$2x = (600)(1)$$

$$x = 300 \text{ min}$$

7.1. Calculating the Rate of Flow

Step 2. Calculate the rate of flow.

Total amount = 200 mL
Administration set = 60 gtt/mL
Running time = 300 min

Using Rule 7.1:

$$\frac{x}{1} = \frac{(200 \text{ mL})(60 \text{ gtt/mL})}{300 \text{ min}}$$

$$300x = (200)(60)$$

$$x = 40 \text{ gtt/min}$$

Answer. Rate of flow = 40 gtt/min

EXAMPLE 7.6

A doctor prescribes a medicated IV solution labeled 250 mg/200 cc. He prescribes 4 mcg/kg/min for a 50-kg patient. If the administration set is 60 gtt/mL, calculate the rate of flow.

Step 1. Calculate the number of mcg per minute for the 50-kg patient.
Since the 50-kg patient is to receive 4 mcg for each kg per min, the number of mcg/kg/min is (4 mcg/kg)(50kg)/min = 200 mcg/min.

Step 2. Calculate the number of minutes the IV should flow.

$$\frac{200 \text{ mcg}}{1 \text{ min}} = \frac{250\,000 \text{ mcg}}{x \text{ min}} \quad \leftarrow 250 \text{ mg}$$

$$200x = (250\,000)(1)$$

$$x = 1250 \text{ min}$$

Step 3. Calculate the rate of flow.

Total amount = 200 mL
Administration set = 60 gtt/mL
Running time = 1250 min

Using Rule 7.1:

$$\frac{x}{1} = \frac{(200 \text{ mL})(60 \text{ gtt/mL})}{1250 \text{ min}}$$

$$1250x = (200)(60)$$

$$x = 9.6 \text{ or } 10 \text{ gtt/min}$$

Answer. Rate of flow = 10 gtt/min

PRACTICE SET 7.1

1. A doctor prescribes glucose 10%, 1000 mL for 10 hours via a 15 gtt/mL delivery system. What is the rate of flow?

2. A physician orders 500 mL of 5% dextrose to run at 150 mL/hr via a 10 gtt/mL administration system. How many gtt/min should the IV drip?

3. Order: 600 mL NS IV for 3 hr via a 15 gtt/mL administration set. What is the rate of flow?

4. Order: 1 L D5LR (dextrose 5% in lactated Ringer's solution) IV for 8 hr via a 20 gtt/mL administration set. What is the rate of flow?

5. Order: 1.5 L D5W (dextrose 5% in water) IV for 360 min. The administration set is a 10 gtt/mL set. Calculate the rate of flow.

6. Order: 1000 mL of 5% dextrose to run at 200 mL/hr. If a microdropper delivery system is used, calculate the rate of flow.

7. Order: 1000 mL NS (normal saline) over 14 hr.
Administration Set: 25 gtt/mL.
Calculate the rate of flow.

8. Order: 75 mL D5W (dextrose 5% in water) over 6 hr.
Administration set: Microdropper administration set.
Calculate the rate of flow.

9. A physician orders 100 mL D5W (dextrose 5% in water) for a child to be administered over 90 min. If the administration set is a microdropper, calculate the rate of flow.

10. A physician orders 1000 mL of D5NS (dextrose 5% in normal saline) for a patient to be given at 100 mL/hr. Calculate the rate of flow if the delivery system is 10 gtt/mL.

11. A patient is to receive 400 mcg/min of an IV medication labeled 400 mg/200 cc. Find the rate of flow if a microdropper administration set is used.

12. An IV mixture is labeled 225 mg/250 cc. The doctor prescribes 3 mcg/kg/min for a 50-kg patient. What is the rate of flow if a microdropper administration set is used?

13. An IV mixture is labeled 200 mg/500 mL. A 154-lb patient is to receive 2 mcg/kg/min via a microdropper administration set. Calculate the rate of flow.

14. A doctor prescribes 200 mL of an IV fluid. If the patient is to receive 5 mL/min via a microdropper administration set, calculate the rate of flow.

7.2 Calculating the Running Time

15. An IV bottle is labeled 12 000 U/250 mL. A 100-lb patient is prescribed 0.2 U/kg/min. Calculate the rate of flow if a microdropper administration set is used.

7.2 CALCULATING THE RUNNING TIME

Sometimes a physician may write an IV order in such a way that the running time is not given. In such a case, you should be able to calculate the running time. Use Rule 7.1, but solve for the running time instead of the rate of flow.

EXAMPLE 7.7

Order: 1000 mL D5LR (dextrose 5% in lactated Ringer's solution) IV. The administration set reads 20 gtt/mL, and the rate of flow is 25 gtt/min. Find the running time.

Total amount = 1000 mL
Administration set = 20 gtt/mL
Rate of flow = 25 gtt/min

Using Rule 7.1:

$$25 \text{ gtt/min} = \frac{(1000 \text{ mL})(20 \text{ gtt/mL})}{x}$$

$$\frac{25}{1} = \frac{(1000)(20)}{x}$$

$$25x = (1000)(20)$$

$$x = 800 \text{ min}$$

Answer. Running time = 800 min or $13\frac{1}{3}$ hr

EXAMPLE 7.8

A small child is given an IV solution of 50 mL of 5% protein hydrolysate, 10 mL of dextrose, and 15 mL of isotonic salt solution at a rate of 100 microdrops per minute via a microdropper administration set. What is the running time?

Total amount = ?
Administration set = 60 gtt/mL
Rate of flow = 100 gtt/min

The total amount of IV fluid to be administered is:

$$\begin{array}{r}50 \text{ mL of 5\% protein hydrolysate} \\ 10 \text{ mL of dextrose} \\ +15 \text{ mL of isotonic salt solution} \\ \hline 75 \text{ mL} \end{array}$$

Using Rule 7.1:

$$100 \text{ gtt/min} = \frac{(75 \text{ mL})(60 \text{ gtt/mL})}{x}$$

$$\frac{100}{1} = \frac{(75)(60)}{x}$$

$$100x = (75)(60)$$

$$x = 45$$

Answer. Running time = 45 min

EXAMPLE 7.9

A doctor orders isotonic sodium lactate 50 mL/kg body mass to be administered intravenously for a 164-lb patient with severe acidosis. The rate of flow is 150 drops/min, and the administration set is 20 gtt/mL. What is the running time?

Total amount = ?
Administration set = 20 gtt/mL
Rate of flow = 150 gtt/min

The total amount to be administered, based on the patient's weight, must be calculated. Divide the problem into three parts.

Part 1. Find the patient's weight in kg.

$$\frac{1 \text{ kg}}{2.2 \text{ lb}} = \frac{x \text{ kg}}{164 \text{ lb}}$$

$$2.2x = (164)(1)$$

$$x = 74.5 \text{ kg}$$

The patient weighs 74.5 kg.

Part 2. Calculate the total amount of sodium lactate needed.

$$\frac{50 \text{ ml}}{1 \text{ kg}} = \frac{x \text{ mL}}{74.5 \text{ kg}}$$

$$1x = (50)(74.5)$$

$$x = 3725 \text{ mL of isotonic sodium lactate}$$

7.2. Calculating the Running Time

Part 3. Solve for the running time.

$$150 \text{ gtt/min} = \frac{(3725 \text{ mL})(20 \text{ gtt/mL})}{x}$$

$$\frac{150}{1} = \frac{(3725)(20)}{x}$$

$$150x = (3725)(20)$$

$$x = 496.67$$

Answer. Running time = 497 min, or about $8\frac{1}{3}$ hr

PRACTICE SET 7.2

1. A small child has been ordered to receive 500 mL of an IV fluid to be run via a microdropper administration set at a rate of 50 gtt/min. What is the running time?

2. A doctor prescribes 3 L of dextran 70 to be run at 100 gtt/min via a 20 gtt/mL administration set. What is the running time?

3. Order: 1 L D5W at 55 gtt/min. If the administration set is 20 gtt/mL, what is the running time?

4. Order: 1.5 L of a normal saline solution at 60 gtt/min. Use a 20 gtt/mL administration system. Calculate the running time.

5. Order: 1000 mL of lactated Ringer's solution (LR) at 25 gtt/min. If a 20 gtt/mL delivery set is used, calculate the running time.

6. Order: 1980 mL LR at 60 gtt/min using a 10 gtt/mL delivery set. Calculate the running time.

7. Calculate the running time for Problem 6 using a 20 gtt/mL delivery system.

8. If a physician orders 1.5 L of dextrose 5% 100 gtt/min via a microdropper administration set, what is the running time?

9. A physician orders 75 mL of 5% protein hydrolysate, 25 mL of dextrose, and 20 mL of isotonic salt solution for a child, to be administered intravenously at the rate of 60 gtt/min via a microdropper administration set. What is the running time?

10. A patient is to receive 2 L dextrose solution via a 15 gtt/mL delivery system. What is the running time if the rate of flow is 60 gtt/min?

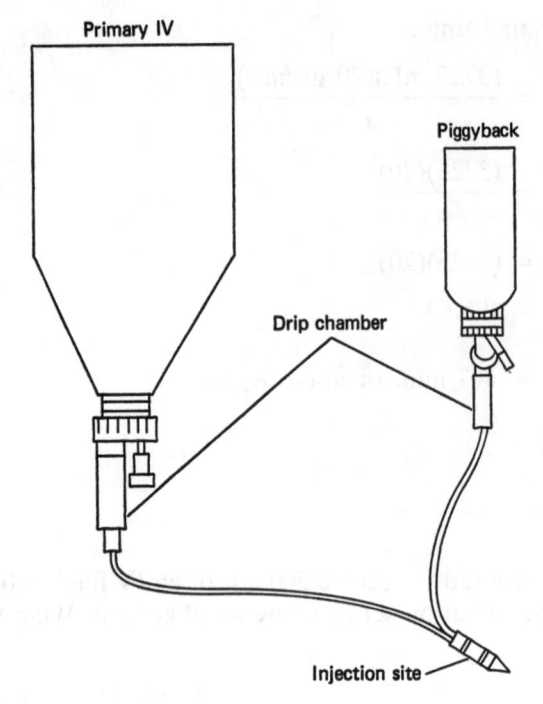

Figure 7-1. Piggyback IV

7.3 PIGGYBACK IVS

Sometimes the drug to be administered is contained in a small bottle to which another larger bottle of solvent is added. This additional small bottle is called an **IV piggyback** (IVPB). The piggyback bottle is usually plugged into the injection site of the primary IV (See Fig. 7-1).

EXAMPLE 7.10

Ampicillin 2 mL in 50 mL NS over 10 minutes is prescribed for a patient suffering from an upper respiratory infection. Calculate the rate of flow if the administration set reads 10 gtt/mL.

Piggyback IV: 2 mL ampicillin
Primary IV: 50 mL NS
IV total: 52 mL

$$\text{Rate of flow} = \frac{(52 \text{ mL})(10 \text{ gtt/mL})}{10 \text{ min}}$$

$$\frac{x}{1} = \frac{(52)(10)}{10}$$

$$x = 52 \text{ gtt/min}$$

Answer. Rate of flow = 52 gtt/min.

7.3. Piggyback IVs

EXAMPLE 7.11

A patient suffering from acute asthma is prescribed 400 mg aminophylline in 50 mL D5W over 1 hr. If the administration set is 15 gtt/mL, calculate the rate of flow. Aminophylline 500 mg/25 mL is available.

Divide the problem into two parts.

Part 1. Solve for the number of mL of aminophylline.

$$\begin{array}{cc} \text{MOH} & = & \text{DM} \\ \downarrow & & \downarrow \end{array}$$

$$\frac{500 \text{ mg}}{25 \text{ mL}} = \frac{400 \text{ mg}}{x \text{ mL}}$$

$$500x = (400)(25)$$

$$x = 20 \text{ mL aminophylline}$$

Calculate amount of IV fluid to be administered.

Piggyback IV: 20 mL aminophylline
Primary IV: 50 mL D5W
IV total: 70 mL

Part 2. Solve for the rate of flow.

$$\text{Rate of flow} = \frac{(70 \text{ mL})(15 \text{ gtt/mL})}{60 \text{ min}}$$

$$\frac{x}{1} = \frac{(70)(15)}{60}$$

$$x = 17.5 \text{ or } 18 \text{ gtt/min}$$

Answer. 18 gtt/min

EXAMPLE 7.12

A physician orders penicillin G potassium 4 000 000 U IV in 100 mL of dextrose to be administered q6h over 1 hr via a 20 gtt/mL administration set. Penicillin G potassium is available in a 5 000 000 U vial. The directions for reconstitution are, "Add 8 mL of sterile water for injection to contents of vial. Resultant solution has a concentration of 500 000 U/mL." Calculate the rate of flow.

Divide the problem into two parts.

Part 1. Calculate the amount of penicillin.

$$\underset{\underset{\dfrac{500\,000\text{ U}}{1\text{ mL}}}{\downarrow}}{\text{MOH}} = \underset{\underset{\dfrac{4\,000\,000\text{ U}}{x\text{ mL}}}{\downarrow}}{\text{DM}}$$

$$500\,000x = (4\,000\,000)(1)$$

$$x = 8\text{ mL}$$

Total amount of IV fluid to be administered.

Piggyback IV: 8 mL penicillin G potassium
Primary IV: 100 mL dextrose
IV total: 108 mL

Part 2. Solve for the rate of flow.

$$\frac{x}{1} = \frac{(108\text{ mL})(20\text{ gtt/mL})}{60\text{ min}}$$

Answer.   Rate of flow = 36 gtt/min

EXAMPLE 7.13

A nurse checked the 10 gtt/mL administration set in a patient's room. 75 mL of D5W was left in the primary IV, and 5 mL of penicillin G potassium was left in the IVPB. If the rate of flow is 10 gtt/min, how long will the bottles last?

Piggyback IV: 5 mL
Primary IV: 75 mL
IV total: 80 mL

Solving for the running time in Rule 7.1:

$$\frac{10\text{ gtt/min}}{1} = \frac{(80\text{ mL})(10\text{ gtt/mL})}{x\text{ min}}$$

$$10x = (80)(10)$$

$$x = 80\text{ min}$$

Answer.   The bottles will last 80 min, or $1\frac{1}{3}$ hr.

PRACTICE SET 7.3

1. Aminophylline 3 mL in 75 mL D5W over 45 minutes is prescribed for a patient suffering from an acute asthma attack. If the administration set is 15 gtt/mL, calculate the rate of flow.

7.4. Chapter 7 Review Problems

2. A physician orders the IV antibiotic ampicillin for a patient suffering from an upper respiratory infection. 500 mg is to be administered intravenously in 50 mL NS over 15 min q6h. If the ampicillin is available after reconstitution as 250 mg/mL, what is the total IV fluid to be administered to the patient? Calculate the rate of flow if the administration set is 15 gtt/mL.

3. Order: Penicillin G potassium 15 000 000 U over 24 hours in 1000 mL of 5% dextrose. Penicillin G potassium is available as 500 000 U/mL. If a 15 gtt/mL administration set is used, calculate the rate of flow.

4. Aminophylline 200 mg in 125 mL 5% dextrose is ordered for an asthma patient. It is to be administered over 2 hr via a 20 gtt/mL administration set. Aminophylline is available 500 mg/20 mL. Calculate the rate of flow.

5. Order: Mandol 1.5 g in 150 mL D5W IV over 1 hr via a 10 gtt/mL delivery system. Mandol is available in a vial, 1 g/100 mL after reconstitution. What is the rate of flow?

6. A nurse saw that a patient's IV administration had suddenly stopped dripping. 150 mL of D5W remained in the primary IV and 25 mL remained in the IVPB. If the 15 gtt/mL administration set had a flow rate of 20 gtt/min, how long would it take to administer the remaining solutions?

7. An IV bottle in a patient's room had 950 cc remaining in it. Because of a malfunction, it was not dripping correctly. If the 15 gtt/mL administration set was calculated to run at a flow rate of 10 gtt/min, how long would the bottle last?

7.4 CHAPTER 7 REVIEW PROBLEMS

1. Order: 5% saline solution 500 mL over 6 hr, IV. Calculate the rate of flow if the administration set is 15 gtt/mL.

2. Order: $\frac{1}{6}$ molar sodium lactate 1200 mL over a 4-hr running time. If the delivery set is a 20 gtt/mL setting, what is the rate of flow?

3. A physician has ordered 1500 mL of isotonic saline to drip 50 drops per minute. How long should the fluid run if the administration set is 15 gtt/mL?

4. A physician has ordered 1000 mL of 3% dextrose to run over a 10-hr period. How many gtt/min should the IV fluid drip if the administration set is 10 gtt/mL?

5. A patient is to be given an IV solution of 45 mL of 5% protein hydrolysate, 10 mL of dextrose, and 15 mL of isotonic salt solution. If, using a micro-

dropper administration set, the rate of flow is 100 microdrops per min, what is the running time?

6. A physician has ordered 2500 mL of 6% dextrose in water to run over a 24-hour period. How many drops per minute should the IV fluid drip if the administration set is 15 gtt/mL?

7. What is the rate of flow for 1.2 L of packed cells IV over 8 hours using equipment with a delivery system of 10 gtt/mL?

8. Order: Glucose 10% 1600 mL/8 hr IV via 15 gtt/mL delivery system. After 4 hr, 600 mL have been delivered. Calculate a new rate in order to finish on time.

9. Order: 100 mL of glucose IV for an infant at 20 microdrops per minute via a microdropper administration set. Calculate the running time.

10. Order: 0.4 g/500 cc mixed IV fluid 400 mcg/min.
Administration set: 20 gtt/mL.
Calculate the rate of flow.

11. Order: IV mixture labeled 0.2 g$\left|\frac{1}{4}\right.$ L for a 187-lb patient; 10 mcg/kg/min.

If the IV solution is to be administered via a 20 gtt/mL delivery set, what is the rate of flow?

12. 600 mL of protein hydrolysate in 600 mL of isotonic salt solution are ordered by a doctor to be administered together at a rate of 25 gtt/min with an administration set of 10 gtt/mL. Calculate the running time.

13. Order: 2000 mL of $\frac{1}{6}$ molar sodium lactate to run at a rate of 150 mL/hr. If the administration set is 25 gtt/mL, how many gtt/min should the IV run?

14. Order: 5% glucose 1000 mL to be administered IV over 8 hours via a 20 gtt/mL delivery system. After 3 hours, 450 mL have been delivered. Calculate a new rate in order to finish on time.

15. Medicated IV Solution: 0.8g/500 cc. An 80-kg patient is to receive 15 mcg/kg/min via a 60 gtt/mL administration set. Calculate the rate of flow.

16. A 100-lb patient is to receive 1.5 L dextrose IV over a period of 10 hr. What would the rate of flow be if the delivery system is 60 gtt/mL?

17. A nurse checked a 10 gtt/mL IV administration set in a patient's room. 375 cc still remained in the IV bottle. If the rate of flow is 12 gtt/min, how long will the bottle last?

18. A patient suffering from severe acidosis has been ordered to receive isotonic sodium lactate 2 L over 15 hr. Calculate the rate of flow using a microdropper delivery system.

19. A patient suffering from asthma has been ordered aminophylline 400 mg qd in 50 mL D5W over 45 minutes. Aminophylline 500 mg/20 mL is available. What is the total amount to be administered, and what is the rate of flow if the delivery set is calibrated 15 gtt/mL?

20. A doctor orders 1 g Mandol in 250 mL 5% dextrose IV q8h over 90 minutes. If, after reconstitution, Mandol is available 1 g/100 mL, what is the total IV solution to be administered q8h? Calculate the rate of flow using a 15 gtt/mL delivery system.

7.5 CHAPTER 7 SELF TEST

7.1 **1.** Order: Dextrose 2 L over 12 hr. The delivery set available has a 15 gtt/mL setting. Calculate the rate of flow.

7.1 **2.** Order: Multiple electrolytes 500 mL in 480 min. If the administration set is 20 gtt/mL, calculate the rate of flow.

7.1 **3.** Order: 600 mL of D5W at 30 gtt/min. If the delivery set is 20 gtt/mL, calculate the running time.

7.2 **4.** Order: 1000 mL D5W at 50 gtt/min. If the administration set is 10 gtt/mL, calculate the running time.

7.1 **5.** Order: Medicated IV fluid 2 g/500 mL. The patient is to receive 1.5 mg/min via a microdropper delivery set. Calculate the rate of flow.

7.1 **6.** What is the rate of flow for 1500 mL of 5% dextrose in water to run at 100 mL/hr if the administration set is 15 gtt/mL?

7.1 **7.** Order: 0.2 U/min of an IV mixture labeled 100 U/200 mL. Administration set: 60 gtt/mL. Calculate the rate of flow.

7.1 **8.** A 120-lb patient is to receive 3.5 L dextrose IV over a period of 18 hr. What is the rate of flow if the administration set is 20 gtt/mL?

7.1 **9.** Glucose 5% 500 mL/4 hr IV via 20 gtt/mL delivery system has been ordered. After 2 hours, 200 mL have been delivered. Calculate a new rate in order to finish on time.

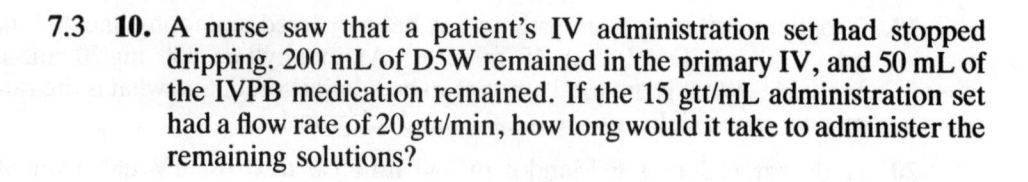

7.3 10. A nurse saw that a patient's IV administration set had stopped dripping. 200 mL of D5W remained in the primary IV, and 50 mL of the IVPB medication remained. If the 15 gtt/mL administration set had a flow rate of 20 gtt/min, how long would it take to administer the remaining solutions?

7.1 11. A doctor prescribes a medicated IV solution labeled 200 mg/250 cc. He prescribes 4 mcg/kg/min for a 70-kg patient. If the administration set is 60 gtt/mL, calculate the rate of flow.

7.3 12. A patient suffering from asthma has been ordered to receive aminophylline 500 mg qd in 75 mL D5W over 1 hr. Aminophylline comes in a 2 g vial. The directions for reconstitution read, "Add 6.8 mL of sterile water for injection to contents of vial. The strength of the resulting solution is 250 mg/mL." If a 20 gtt/mL delivery set is used, calculate the rate of flow.

7.3 13. 0.5 L of protein hydrolysate in 0.5 L NS has been ordered to be administered intravenously to a patient. If the rate of flow is 20 gtt/min, and if the administration set is 10 gtt/mL, calculate the running time.

7.2 14. How long should an IV run for an infant who has been prescribed 100 mL of glucose to be administered at the rate of 50 gtt/min via a microdropper administration set?

7.1 15. A patient is to receive $1\frac{1}{4}$ liters of dextrose over a period of 10 hr via a microdropper administration set. Calculate the rate of flow.

SUMMARY OF CHAPTER 7 RULES

RULE 7.1 Rule for Calculating the Rate of Flow for IV Fluids

$$\text{Rate of flow} = \frac{(\text{Amount of fluid})(\text{Administration set calibration})}{\text{Running time}}$$

$$\frac{x}{1} = \frac{(\text{mL})(\text{gtt/mL})}{\text{min}}$$

8
Calculations for Pediatric Dosages

OBJECTIVES

After studying this chapter you should be able to

1. calculate pediatric dosages;
2. work practical problems involving pediatric medications.

INTRODUCTION

Infants and children do not receive the same amount of medication as do adults. In treating a child, you should not consider the child as a miniature adult, but as a unique person who requires special attention. Even though a doctor prescribes the medication for children, you are responsible for knowing what constitutes the safe range of pediatric dosages. Various rules have been devised for the calculation of pediatric dosages.

8.1 CALCULATING PEDIATRIC DOSAGES BASED ON BODY SURFACE

The most accurate way of determining the correct pediatric dosage is by using the child's size calculated in terms of body surface area. The body surface of a child is measured in m^2. If a child's body surface area is given, the Surface Area

Rule 8.1 can be used immediately. The 1.73 m² stated in the denominator of the fraction is the accepted average adult body surface area.

RULE 8.1 Surface Area Rule

$$\text{Child's dose} = \frac{(\text{Surface area in m}^2)(\text{Adult dose})}{1.73 \text{ m}^2}$$

EXAMPLE 8.1

The adult dose for Demerol is 50 mg. A child with a body surface of 0.6 m² should receive how much Demerol?

Surface area = 0.6 m²
Adult dose = 50 mg

Using Rule 8.1:

$$\text{Child's dose} = \frac{(0.6 \text{ m}^2)(50 \text{ mg})}{1.73 \text{ m}^2}$$

Answer. Child's dose = 17.3 mg Demerol

EXAMPLE 8.2

How many mg Garamycin should an infant with a body surface of 0.2 m² receive if the adult dose is 60 mg?

Surface area = 0.2 m²
Adult dose = 60 mg

Using Rule 8.1:

$$\text{Child's dose} = \frac{(0.2 \text{ m}^2)(60 \text{ mg})}{1.73 \text{ m}^2}$$

Answer. Child's dose = 6.9 mg Garamycin

Sometimes a child's body surface area is not given. If this is the case, you can calculate a child's body surface area using a West Nomogram, a chart that relates a child's height and weight in terms of the body surface. (See Appendix III.) The enclosed column estimates the body surface of children of average build using weight alone.

Body surface areas can be calculated using Rule 8.2.

8.1. Calculating Pediatric Dosages Based on Body Surface

RULE 8.2 Rule for Reading the West Nomogram

Step 1. Find the height (in either cm or in.) of the child in the height column.

Step 2. Find the weight (in either kg or lb) of the child in the weight column.

Step 3. Draw a straight line connecting the height point and the weight point of the child. The number where the line intersects the surface-area column is the child's body surface area.

EXAMPLE 8.3

Calculate the body surface area of a child who is 35 in. tall and who weighs 28 lb.

Step 1. Find the child's height, 35 in., in the height column.

Step 2. Find the child's weight, 28 lb, in the weight column.

Step 3. Draw a straight line connecting the 35-in. point with the 28-lb point. The line intersects the surface-area column at 0.57 m^2.

Answer. The child's surface area is 0.57 m^2.

The three steps are illustrated in Figure 8–1. Usually, surface area can be read to the nearest hundredth.

EXAMPLE 8.4

Calculate the body surface area of a child whose height is 82 cm and who weighs 12 kg.

The steps to solve this problem are illustrated in Figure 8–2.

Answer. The body surface area is 0.53 m^2.

It is the point where the straight line intersects the surface-area column.

EXAMPLE 8.5

A child who weighs 26 kg and who is 111 cm tall has been prescribed atropine sulfate. The usual adult dose is 0.4 mg. How many mg should the child receive?

Step 1. Find the body surface area of the child using the West Nomogram. Reading the Nomogram, the body surface area of the child is 0.90 m^2.

Step 2. Use the surface area rule to calculate the child's dose.

$$\text{Child's dose} = \frac{0.90 \text{ m}^2 \times 0.4 \text{ mg}}{1.73 \text{ m}^2}$$

Answer. Child's dose = 0.2 mg atropine sulfate.

180 8. Calculations for Pediatric Dosages

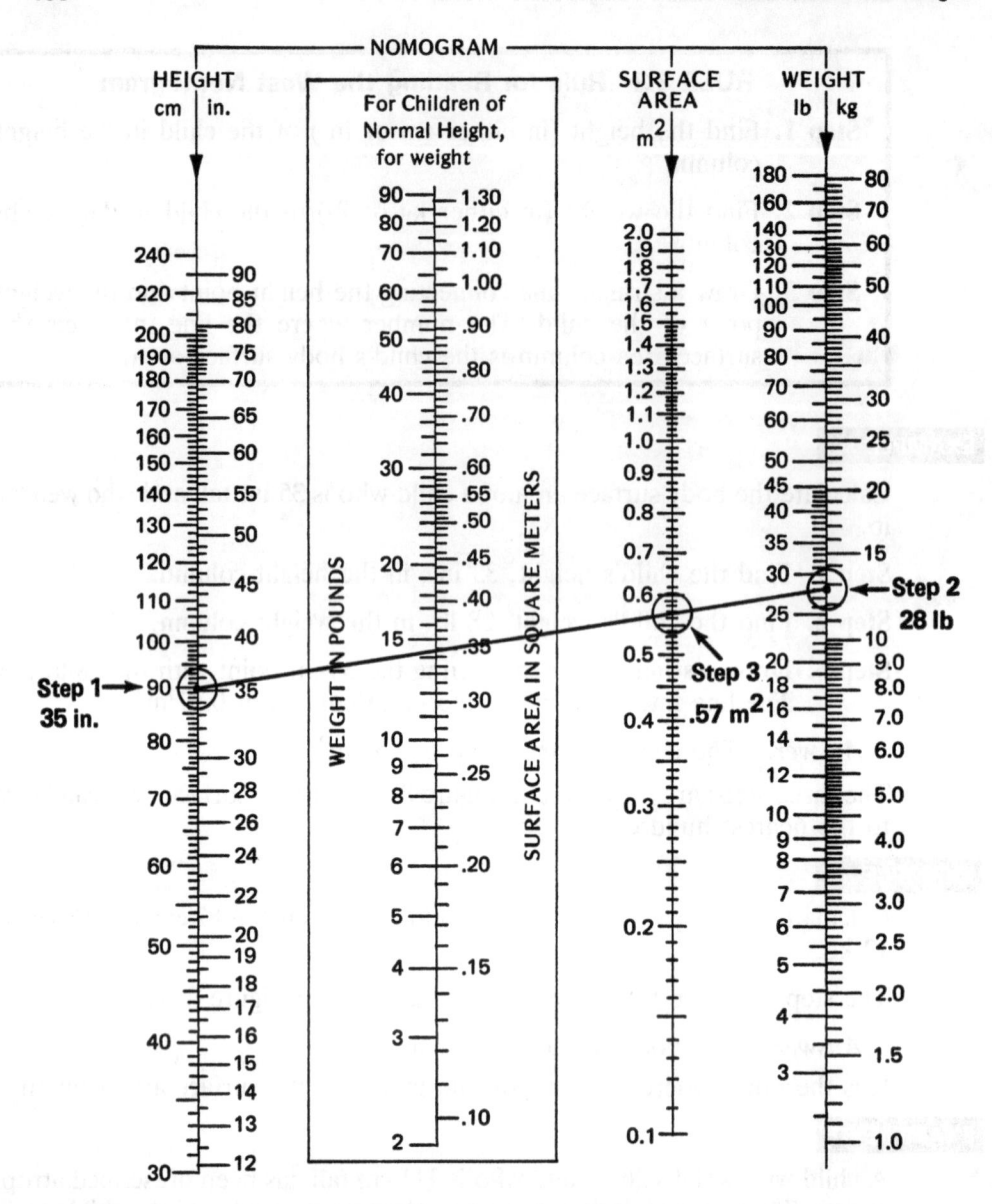

Figure 8–1. West Nomogram

EXAMPLE 8.6

Calculate the dosage of a sulfa drug for a child who is 24 in. tall and who weighs 35 lb. The sulfa drug order calls for 2 g/m² body surface for the child.

Step 1. The child's surface area must be calculated. Using the West Nomogram, the body surface is 0.56 m².

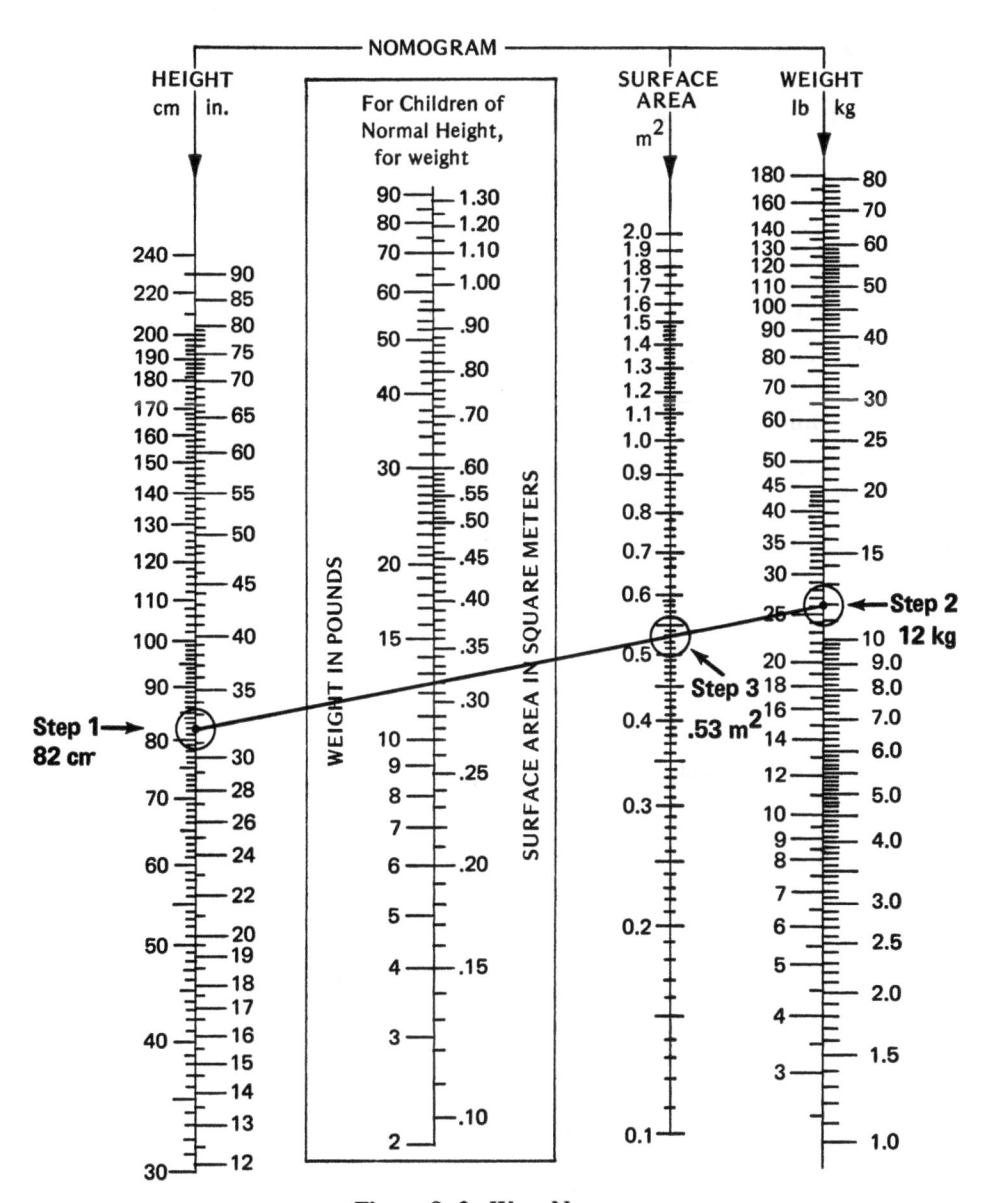

8.1. Calculating Pediatric Dosages Based on Body Surface

Figure 8-2. West Nomogram

Step 2. Solve for the amount of sulfa drug for the child based on the drug order. The drug order calls for 2 g/m².

$$\frac{2\text{g}}{1\text{ m}^2} = \frac{x \text{ g}}{0.56 \text{ m}^2}$$

$$x = (2)(0.56)$$

$$x = 1.1 \text{ g}$$

Answer. The child's dose is 1.1 g of the sulfa drug.

PRACTICE SET 8.1

1. The adult dose of Demerol is 50 mg. Calculate the child's dose of Demerol for a child with a body surface of 0.45 m^2.

2. An adult receives gr x of aspirin. How many gr should be given to a child who is 96 cm tall and who weighs 16 kg?

3. A doctor has prescribed tetracycline for a child who weighs 26 lb and who is 34 in. tall. The usual adult dose of tetracycline is 50 mg. Calculate the child's dose.

4. Calculate the surface area for a child who is 18.5 in. tall and who weighs 8 lb.

5. The adult dose of atropine is gr $\frac{1}{150}$. Calculate the correct dose for a child who has a body surface of 0.86 m^2.

6. Adult dose: Atarax 25 mg
   Child's body mass: 10 lb
   Child's height: 22 in.
   Solve for the child's dose.

7. Calculate the child's dose of sulfisoxazole for a child who weighs 57 kg and is 100 cm tall. The order is for 2 g/m^2 body surface for the child.

8. Doctor's order: Epinephrine, 300 mcg/m^2
   Child's height: 50 in.
   Child's body mass: 50 lb
   Calculate the correct pediatric dosage.

9. Child's height: 105 cm
   Child's body mass: 20 kg
   Calculate the body surface area of the child.

10. Calculate the dosage in *mg* of chloral hydrate for a child who is 42 in. tall and weighs 50 lb. The prescription calls for 0.2 g/m^2.

8.2 CALCULATING PEDIATRIC DOSAGES BASED ON AGE AND BODY MASS

There are other rules dealing with a child's age and body mass that are used to calculate pediatric dosages. Although these rules are seldom used, you should be familiar with them.

8.2. Calculating Pediatric Dosages Based on Age and Body Mass

> **RULE 8.3 Fried's Rule (Birth to 12 months)**
>
> $$\text{Infant's dose} = \frac{(\text{Age in months})(\text{Adult dose})}{150}$$

> **RULE 8.4 Young's Rule (1–12 years)**
>
> $$\text{Child's dose} = \frac{(\text{Age in yr})(\text{Adult dose})}{\text{Age in yr} + 12}$$

> **RULE 8.5 Clark's Rule**
>
> $$\text{Child's dose} = \frac{(\text{Mass of child})(\text{Adult dose})}{150 \text{ lb or } 68 \text{ kg}}$$

EXAMPLE 8.7

How many cc of castor oil would be given to a 10-month-old infant if the adult dose is 15 cc?

Infant's age = 10 months
Adult dose = 15 cc

Using Rule 8.3:

$$\text{Infant's dose} = \frac{(10 \text{ months})(15 \text{ cc})}{150}$$

Infant's dose = 1 cc castor oil

EXAMPLE 8.8

If the adult dose of a drug is gr $\frac{1}{4}$, what is the dose for a 10-year-old boy?

Child's age = 10 yr
Child's age + 12 = 22 yr
Adult dose = gr $\frac{1}{4}$ = 0.25 gr

$$\text{Child's dose} = \frac{(10 \text{ yr})(0.25 \text{ gr})}{22 \text{ yr}}$$

Child's dose = 0.1 gr of the drug

EXAMPLE 8.9

The adult dose of Keflin is 100 mg. What is the dose for a child weighing 50 lb?

Child's mass in lb = 50 lb
Adult dose = 100 mg

Using Rule 8.5:

$$\text{Child's dose} = \frac{(50 \text{ lb})(100 \text{ mg})}{150 \text{ lb}}$$

Child's dose = 33.3 mg Keflin

EXAMPLE 8.10

A 44-kg child has been ordered to receive a dose of cortisone acetate. If the adult dose is 150 mg, what will the child's dose be?

Child's mass in kg = 44 kg
Adult's dose = 150 mg

Using Rule 8.5:

$$\text{Child's dose} = \frac{(44 \text{ kg})(150 \text{ mg})}{68 \text{ kg}}$$

Child's dose = 97.1 mg cortisone acetate

PRACTICE SET 8.2

1. The adult dose for penicillin is 300 000 U. How many units should you administer to a 45-lb child?

2. An adult dose for phenobarbital is 30 mg. How many mg should a 10-year-old child receive?

3. An 11-month-old child has been prescribed Demerol. How many mg should the infant receive if the adult dose is 75 mg?

4. If the adult dose of Fowler's solution is ℳ iii, how many minims would be administered to a 6-year-old child?

5. How much tincture of digitalis would you administer to a 17-kg child if the adult dose is 1 mL?

6. If the adult dose of phenobarbital is 30 mg, what is the dosage for a 6-month-old infant?

7. What dose of Vitamin K will you give to a 12-year-old child if the adult dose is 2 mg?
8. A doctor has ordered Milk of Magnesia for a 7-month-old infant. What is the correct dosage if the adult dose is 30 mL?
9. A child weighs 37 kg. A doctor prescribes Tempra. If the adult dose is 325 mg, how many mg will be administered to the child?
10. If an adult dose of a drug is 600 mg, what is the dose for an 8-year-old child?

8.3 CHAPTER 8 REVIEW PROBLEMS

1. The adult dose of phenobarbital is 30 mg. How much should a 3-year-old child receive?
2. Order: Keflin. The adult dosage is 100 mg. What is the dosage for a child with a surface area of 1.5 m^2?
3. If the adult dosage of tincture of digitalis is ℳ xii, what is the dosage for a 6-year-old child?
4. The adult dose for adrenalin is 10 mg. What is the dose of adrenalin for a child weighing 45 lb?
5. The adult dose for morphine is 5 mg. How much morphine should a 6-month-old child receive?
6. Calculate the dosage of chloral hydrate for a child who is 45 in. tall and who weighs 50 lb. The usual adult dosage is 200 mg.
7. The adult dose of atropine sulfate is gr $\frac{1}{150}$. What is the dose for a 30-month-old child?
8. The adult dose for Nembutal is 90 mg. What dose would be administered to a 9-month-old infant?
9. A child weighs 75 lb. If the adult dosage of sulfadiazine is 500 mg, what is the dosage for this child?
10. Child's height: 55 in.
    Child's body mass: 75 lb
    Calculate the child's surface area.
11. The adult dose of erythromycin is 250 mg. Calculate the correct pediatric dosage for a child who weighs 28 kg.

12. The adult dose of castor oil is 15 cc. How much should be administered to a 10-month-old child?

13. The doctor prescribes epinephrine 5 mg/m^2 for a child. Calculate the mg for a child who is 85 cm tall and has 6.4 kg body mass.

14. Calculate the correct dosage of penicillin for a child with a body surface of 0.72 m^2 if the average adult dose is 300 000 U.

15. The order of hydrocodone bitartrate is 20 mg/m^2. If a child is 106 cm tall and weighs 21 kg, calculate the amount of hydrocodone bitartrate for the child.

8.4 CHAPTER 8 SELF TEST

8.2 1. What is the dose in mg of adrenalin for a child weighing 17 kg if the adult dose is 1 mg?

8.2 2. A 10-month-old infant has been prescribed Gantrisin. If the adult dose is 800 mg, how many mg should you give the infant?

8.2 3. The adult dose of penicillin is 400 000 U. How much should a 5-year-old child receive?

8.1 4. Order: Epinephrine 200 mcg/m^2 body surface for a child who is 70 cm tall and who weighs 12 kg. How many mcg should you administer?

8.1 5. The adult dose of atropine is gr iii. What is the dose in gr for an infant with 0.25 m^2 body surface area?

8.1 6. Child's height: 64 in.
Child's body mass: 95 lb
Calculate the child's body surface area.

8.2 7. A doctor prescribes Milk of Magnesia for a 5-month-old child. The usual adult dose is 30 mL. Calculate the correct pediatric dose.

8.2 **8.** Order: Demerol
Adult dose: 120 mg
Calculate the correct dose for a $4\frac{1}{2}$-year-old child.

8.2 **9.** A child has a body mass of 75 lb. If the adult dose for Cleocin is 200 mg, how much Cleocin should the child receive?

8.1 **10.** A doctor prescribes sulfisoxazole 2 g/m² for a child who is 34 in. tall and who weighs 30 lb. Calculate the correct pediatric dosage for this child.

8.1 **11.** The surface area of a child is 1 m². Calculate the correct pediatric dosage of ampicillin if the adult dose is 250 mg.

8.2 **12.** Order: Nembutal
Adult dose: 90 mg
Calculate the correct dose for a 3-month-old infant

8.2 **13.** If the adult dose of a drug is gr $\frac{1}{4}$, calculate the dose for a 10-year-old child.

8.2 **14.** The adult dosage of Dramamine is 50 mg. Calculate the correct dose for a 60-lb child.

8.1 **15.** The adult dose of paregoric is 10 mL. Calculate the correct dosage for a child who weighs 60 kg and who is 122 cm tall.

SUMMARY OF CHAPTER 8 RULES

RULE 8.1   Surface Area Rule

$$\text{Child's dose} = \frac{(\text{Surface area in m}^2)(\text{Adult dose})}{1.73 \text{ m}^2}$$

RULE 8.2 Rule for Reading the West Nomogram

Step 1. Find the height (in either cm or in.) of the child in the height column.

Step 2. Find the weight (in either kg or lb) of the child in the weight column.

Step 3. Draw a straight line connecting the height point and the weight point of the child. The number where the line intersects the surface-area column is the child's body surface area.

RULE 8.3 Fried's Rule (Birth to 12 months)

$$\text{Infant's dose} = \frac{(\text{Age in months})(\text{Adult dose})}{150}$$

RULE 8.4 Young's Rule (1–12 years)

$$\text{Child's dose} = \frac{(\text{Age in yr})(\text{Adult dose})}{\text{Age in yr} + 12}$$

RULE 8.5 Clark's Rule

$$\text{Child's dose} = \frac{(\text{Mass of child})(\text{Adult dose})}{150 \text{ lb or } 68 \text{ kg}}$$

9
Computer-Generated Medication Administration Records

OBJECTIVES

After studying this chapter you should be able to

1. read the time from a twenty-four-hour clock;
2. write the time of day using the twenty-four-hour clock;
3. interpret orders from computer-generated medication administration records.

INTRODUCTION

Record keeping is becoming an enormous and time-consuming job in hospitals. The valuable time of the nurse is often taken up by the minute and detailed entries needed to keep a patient's medical record accurate and up-to-date. For this reason, many hospitals are converting to computers for processing their drug orders. A patient's drug order is entered into the computer from the physician's order form. This is forwarded to the pharmacy, after which a computer-generated medication sheet listing all the ordered drugs for a patient is sent, daily, to the patient's nursing unit.

With this computerized system, the hospital pharmacist can always delete the drugs that have been discontinued, as well as add any new drugs prescribed by the physician. The hospital computer may also have the capability of scanning the entered data for drug incompatabilities, drug allergies, safe dosage ranges, and administration times.

What is significant for the nurse is that the medication administration record (MAR) may be printed directly from the computer. Therefore, it is important that the nurse be able to interpret a computer-generated medication administration record. Included on the computer printout will be all of the patient's medications, their dosage, frequency of administration, route, and times of administration.

Not all computer-generated printouts for the medication administration records are the same. Several examples will be illustrated in this chapter so that you will at least have a general knowledge of computer-generated medication administration records.

9.1 TWENTY-FOUR-HOUR CLOCK

Many hospitals have converted traditional clock time into twenty-four-hour clock time. Computer-generated medication administration records usually use the twenty-four-hour clock when denoting administration times. Therefore, it is imperative that you learn to read and write the time using the twenty-four-hour clock.

Table 9.1 shows equivalent times of the traditional clock with which you are familiar, and the twenty-four-hour clock.

Notice that the twenty-four-hour clock uses four digits. 1:00 A.M. through 9:00 A.M. have the same last three digits on both clocks, but, on the twenty-four-hour clock, they also have a zero for the first digit. 10:00 A.M., 11:00 A.M., and 12:00 P.M. have the same four digits on both clocks. The difference between the clocks essentially occurs from 1:00 P.M. to 12:00 A.M. 1:00 P.M. becomes 1300 (12:00 + 1:00 = 1300), 2:00 P.M. becomes 1400 (12:00 + 2:00 = 1400), and so on. This is the pattern for all the rest of the hours on the twenty-four-hour clock.

EXAMPLE 9.1

Convert 5:00 P.M. to 24-hour clock time.

Add: 12:00 + 5:00
    12:00 + 5:00 = 17:00 = 1700

Answer. 5:00 P.M. = 1700

EXAMPLE 9.2

Convert 11:00 P.M. to 24-hour clock time.

Add: 12:00 + 11:00
    12:00 + 11:00 = 23:00 = 2300

9.1. Twenty-four-Hour Clock

TABLE 9–1 TWENTY-FOUR-HOUR CLOCK

Traditional Clock	24-Hour Clock
1:00 A.M.	0100
2:00 A.M.	0200
3:00 A.M.	0300
4:00 A.M.	0400
5:00 A.M.	0500
6:00 A.M.	0600
7:00 A.M.	0700
8:00 A.M.	0800
9:00 A.M.	0900
10:00 A.M.	1000
11:00 A.M.	1100
12:00 P.M.	1200
1:00 P.M.	1300
2:00 P.M.	1400
3:00 P.M.	1500
4:00 P.M.	1600
5:00 P.M.	1700
6:00 P.M.	1800
7:00 P.M.	1900
8:00 P.M.	2000
9:00 P.M.	2100
10:00 P.M.	2200
11:00 P.M.	2300
12:00 A.M.	2400

Answer. 11:00 P.M. = 2300

EXAMPLE 9.3

Convert 1500 to traditional clock time.

Subtract: 1500 − 1200
1500 − 1200 = 0300 = 3:00 P.M.

Answer. 1500 = 3:00 P.M.

EXAMPLE 9.4

Convert 2400 to traditional clock time.

Subtract: 2400 − 1200
2400 − 1200 = 1200 = 12:00 A.M.

Answer. 2400 = 12:00 A.M.

PRACTICE SET 9.1

Convert each of the traditional clock times to twenty-four-hour clock time.
1. 1:00 A.M.
2. 2:00 P.M.
3. 6:00 P.M.
4. 11:00 A.M.
5. 1:00 P.M.
6. 11:00 P.M.
7. 5:00 A.M.
8. 9:00 P.M.
9. 12:00 A.M.
10. 8:00 P.M.
11. 6:00 A.M.
12. 12:00 P.M.
13. 3:00 P.M.
14. 2:00 A.M.
15. 10:00 P.M.

Convert each of the twenty-four-hour clock times to traditional clock time.
16. 2100
17. 0200
18. 0700
19. 1300
20. 0100
21. 1600
22. 2000
23. 1500
24. 0500
25. 1800

26. 0800

27. 2400

28. 1900

29. 1700

30. 1400

9.2 COMPUTER-GENERATED MEDICATION ADMINISTRATION RECORDS

Even though each hospital has a computer program used to generate its own unique medication administration records, there are some common data in all of them. The main data to be recognized by the nurse on a printout are these:

1. Name of the patient
2. Date and time when order was written
3. Name of the drug to be administered
4. Dosage of the drug
5. Route by which the drug is to be administered
6. Time and/or frequency of administration
7. Specific instructions or notations about the medications

Typical computer-generated medication administration records are illustrated in the following figures.

NO	MEDICATION DOSE, FREQUENCY
SCH 12	DSS 250 MG CAP– 1 CAP BID PO
PRN 5	VICODIN (HYDROCODONE/APAP) TAB 1 TAB Q4H PRN PAIN, PRN PO HEADACHE

Figure 9–1. Medication administration record

1. Number column (See Fig. 9–1)

   a. Medications are determined by the Pharmacy as SCH or PRN. SCH means that medication is administered on a schedule. PRN means that medication is administered as needed.

b. The number beneath SCH or PRN is the random number assigned by the pharmacy as a prescription number. This number can be used by the nurse when referring the medication to the pharmacist. This number should not be confused with the medication dosage.

MEDICATION RECORD | NOTE:

ADMINISTRATION PERIOD 07:01 03/13/87 to 07:00 03/14/87				A.M. SHIFT	P.M. SHIFT	NOC SHIFT
NO	MEDICATION DOSE, FREQUENCY	START DATE	STOP DATE	0701 to 1500	1501 to 2300	2301 to 0700
SCH 2	DURICEF (CEFADROXIL) 500 MG CAP– 1 GRAM BID PO	03/12/87		09:00	21:00	
		RENEW 03/16/87				

Figure 9–2. Medication administration record

2. First line (See Fig. 9–2)

   The first line lists the trade or proprietary name of the medication followed in parenthesis by the generic name. After the medication name, the pharmacist lists the dose as supplied by the pharmacy.

MEDICATION RECORD | NOTE:

ADMINISTRATION PERIOD 06:00 06/02/87 to 05:59 06/03/87				A.M. SHIFT	P.M. SHIFT	NOC SHIFT
NO	MEDICATION DOSE, FREQUENCY	START DATE	STOP DATE	0701 to 1500	1501 to 2300	2301 to 0700
SCH 1	DESYREL (TRAZODONE) 50 MG TAB– 1/2 TAB = 25 MG BID* PO	06/01/87		09:00	18:00	
		RENEW				
SCH 1	DESYREL (TRAZODONE) 50 MG TAB– 1&1/2 TAB = 75 MG HS PO	06/01/87			22:00	
		RENEW				

Figure 9–3. Medication administration record

3. Second line (See Fig. 9–3)

   a. The second line lists the dose prescribed by the physician.

   b. For medications that have a different dose prescribed according to the hour of administration, the medication will have multiple entries. The hour of medication is printed respectively on the shift(s) it is to be given.

9.2. Computer-Generated Medication Administration Records

4. Third line (see Fig. 9-4)

    The third line lists specific instructions or notations about the medication.

5. Start/Stop/Renew Date (See Fig 9-4)

    These dates indicate when the medication is to be started, stopped, or renewed.

MEDICATION RECORD | NOTE:

ADMINISTRATION PERIOD 07:01 05/21/87 to 07:00 05/22/87

NO	MEDICATION DOSE, FREQUENCY	START DATE	STOP DATE
SCH 8	TONOCARD (TOCAINIDE) 400 MG TAB– 1 TAB TIDPC PO	05/20/87	
		RENEW	
SCH 9	TRANSDERM-NITRO 5 MG 1 PATCH QD TDP AT HS	05/20/87	
		RENEW	
SCH 10	LANOXIN (DIGOXIN) 0.125 MG TAB– 1 TAB QD1300 CHECK PULSE	05/20/87	
		RENEW	

Figure 9-4. Medication administration record

Usually, a licensed nurse is assigned to check the accuracy of the daily MAR, but it is each nurse's responsibility to interpret each patient's MAR and administer the correct medication dosage.

EXAMPLE 9.5

Referring to the MAR in Figure 9-5 (on page 196), answer the following questions:

(a) Which medications should be given as scheduled?

   Answer. Heparin and DSS

(b) Which medications should be given as needed for pain?

   Answer. Meperidine, Vistaril, Vicodin, and Dulcolax

(c) Which medication has a prescription identification number of 9?

   Answer. Vistaril

MEDICATION RECORD | NOTE:

ADMINISTRATION PERIOD 07:01 03/13/87 to 07:00 03/14/87

NO	MEDICATION DOSE, FREQUENCY	START DATE	STOP DATE
SCH 7	HEPARIN LOCK 100 U/1ML 1 VIAL Q6H IV	03/12/87 RENEW	
SCH 11	DSS 250 MG CAP– 1 CAP BID PO	03/12/87 RENEW	
IIV 3	CEFAZOLIN .... 1 GRAM D5W .... 50 ML X3 DAYS Q6H	03/10/87 RENEW 03/14/87	03/14/87
PRN 1	MEPERIDINE 50MG/1ML AMP 25-50 MG Q4H PRN PRN IM GIVE WITH VISTARIL	03/09/87 RENEW 03/13/87	
PRN 9	VISTARIL (HYDROXYZINE) 100 MG INJ 25 MG Q4H PRN IM GIVE WITH DEMEROL	03/12/87 RENEW	
PRN 10	VICODIN (HYDROCODONE/APAP) TAB 1 TAB Q4H FOR PAIN PRN PO	03/12/87 RENEW	
PRN 12	DUCOLAX (BISACODYL) 5 MG TAB 2 TAB PRN CONSTIPAT– PRN PO ION	03/12/87 RENEW	

Figure 9–5. Medication administration record

(d) Which medication started on March 9, 1987?

Answer. Meperidine

(e) Which medication was renewed on March 14, 1987?

Answer. Cefazolin

(f) What are the special instructions given for meperidine?

Answer. Give with Vistaril

(g) What is the generic name for Dulcolax?

Answer. Bisacodyl

9.2. Computer-Generated Medication Administration Records

(h) What is the generic name for Vistaril?

Answer. Hydroxyzine

(i) What is the dosage of Vistaril prescribed by the physician?

Answer. 25 mg q4h

(j) What is the dosage of Dulcolax supplied by the pharmacy?

Answer. 5 mg tablets

(k) What is the dosage of meperidine prescribed by the physician?

Answer. 25–50 mg q4h prn

(l) How many mg of Dulcolax does the physician prescribe per dose?

Answer. 10 mg

(m) How many mL would you administer to the patient if you administered 25 mg of meperidine?

Answer. 0.5 mL

EXAMPLE 9.6

Figure 9–6 illustrates a computer-generated medication administration record from a different hospital.

ALLERGIES:					
MEDICATION	GENERIC NAME DESCRIPTION	(TRADE NAME)	2300–0700	0700–1500	1500–2300
DATE Rx#	COMMENTS	ROUTE FREQ.	(11–7)	(7–3)	(3–11)
MEPERIDINE 1 MG IM Q03 HRS PRN 09-15 006 75 MG/ML INJ		DEMEROL			
ACETAMINOPHEN/CODEINE 1 TAB PO Q04 HRS PRN 09-15 088 325 MG TABLET W/ 30 MG CODEINE		TYLENOL #3			

Figure 9–6. Medication administration record

The first line lists the medication's generic name and its trade name. The second line lists the required medication dosage as well as the route and frequency of the administration as prescribed by the physician. The last line lists the date, the prescription number, and the dosage, as supplied by the pharmacy.

(a) What is the trade name for meperidine?

Answer. Demerol

(b) What is the dosage of acetaminophen/codeine as supplied by the pharmacy?

Answer. 325 mg tablet acetaminophen with 30 mg codeine

(c) By what route should meperidine be administered to the patient?

Answer. By injection into the muscle

(d) What is the date of the medication administration record?

Answer. September 15

PRACTICE SET 9.2

Use the MAR illustrated in Figure 9–7 for questions 1 through 7.

1. What is the generic name for Aldomet?
2. What was the start date for Isosorbide?
3. At what times should Aldomet be administered? Give the answer in traditional clock time.

MEDICATION RECORD | NOTE:

ADMINISTRATION PERIOD 07:01 03/13/87 to 07:00 03/14/87				A.M. SHIFT	P.M. SHIFT	NOC SHIFT
NO	MEDICATION DOSE, FREQUENCY	START DATE	STOP DATE	0701 to 1500	1501 to 2300	2301 to 0700
SCH 1	ALDOMET (METHYLDOPA) 250 MG TAB– 1 TAB TID PO	03/12/87		09:00 13:00	17:00	
		RENEW				
SCH 5	ISOSORBIDE 5 MG ORAL TAB– 1 TAB TID PO	03/12/87		09:00 13:00	17:00	
		RENEW				

Figure 9–7. Medication administration record

9.2. Computer-Generated Medication Administration Records

4. What is the prescription identification number for Isosorbide?

5. How many mg of Aldomet should be administered to the patient per dose?

6. What is the dose of Isosorbide supplied by the pharmacy?

7. Is there a renewal date for either medication?

Use the MAR illustrated in Figure 9-8 for questions 8 through 15.

MEDICATION RECORD | NOTE:

ADMINISTRATION PERIOD 06:00 06/02/87 to 05:59 06/03/87			A.M. SHIFT	P.M. SHIFT	NOC SHIFT
NO	MEDICATION DOSE, FREQUENCY	START DATE / STOP DATE	0701 to 1500	1501 to 2300	2301 to 0700
SCH 1	DESYREL (TRAZODONE) 50 MG TAB– 1/2 TAB = 25 MG BID* PO	06/01/87 / RENEW	09:00	18:00	
SCH 2	DESYREL (TRAZODONE) 50 MG TAB– 1&1/2 TAB = 75 MG HS PO	06/01/87 / RENEW		22:00	

Figure 9-8. Medication administration record

8. What is the generic name for Desyrel?

9. At what times (traditional clock time) should 25 mg of Desyrel be administered?

10. At what time (traditional clock time) should 75 mg of Desyrel be administered?

11. What is the dose of Desyrel supplied by the pharmacy?

12. What was the start date for administering Desyrel?

13. How many tablets of Desyrel should be administered at 10:00 P.M.?

14. Is this medication administered as necessary for pain?

15. How many mg of Desyrel should be administered at 6:00 P.M.?

Use the MAR illustrated in Figure 9-9 (on page 200) for questions 16 through 20.

16. What is the trade name for acetaminophen?

17. How often can acetaminophen be administered to the patient?

ALLERGIES:					
MEDICATION DATE Rx#	GENERIC NAME DESCRIPTION COMMENTS	(TRADE NAME) ROUTE FREQ.	2300–0700 (11–7)	0700–1500 (7–3)	1500–2300 (3–11)
09-15 004 1,000 MG INJ	CEFAZOLIN 1 MG IV Q06H	ANCEF			
09-15 009 325 MG TABLET	ACETAMINOPHEN 2 TABS PO Q 4 HRS PRN	ANACIN-3			

Figure 9–9. Medication administration record

18. What is the route of administration for cefazolin?

19. How often should cefazolin be administered?

20. What strength tablet of acetaminophen is supplied by the pharmacy?

9.3 CHAPTER 9 REVIEW PROBLEMS

Convert the traditional clock time to twenty-four-hour clock time.

1. 2:00 P.M.

2. 7:00 P.M.

3. 12:00 P.M.

4. 9:00 A.M.

5. 11:00 P.M.

Convert the twenty-four-hour clock time to traditional time.

6. 2200

7. 0300

8. 1700

9. 1300

10. 2000

Use the MAR illustrated in Figure 9–10 to answer questions 11 through 20.

11. What is the generic name for Tonocard?

MEDICATION RECORD | NOTE:

ADMINISTRATION PERIOD 07:01 05/21/87 to 07:00 05/22/87

NO	MEDICATION DOSE, FREQUENCY	START DATE	STOP DATE
SCH 8	TONOCARD (TOCAINIDE) 400 MG TAB– 1 TAB TIDPC PO	05/20/87 RENEW	
SCH 9	TRANSDERM-NITRO 5 MG 1 PATCH QD TDP AT HS	05/20/87 RENEW	
PRN 1	VICODIN (HYDROCODONE/APAP) TAB 1 TAB Q4H PRN PAIN PRN PO	05/20/87 RENEW	
PRN 5	BENADRYL (DIPHENHYDRAMINE) 50MG INJ 50MG Q8H PRN PRN INJ	05/20/87 RENEW	

Figure 9–10. Medication administration record

12. What strength tablet of Benadryl is supplied by the pharmacy?
13. By what route and how often can Benadryl be administered?
14. How often can Vicodin be administered to the patient?
15. How many mg of Benadryl should be administered per dose?
16. What is the generic name for Benadryl?
17. How many mg of Tonocard should be administered per dose?
18. What is the prescription number for Tonocard?
19. Which medications are scheduled medications?
20. What is the prescription number for Benadryl?

9.4 CHAPTER 9 SELF TEST

Convert the traditional clock time to twenty-four-hour clock time.

9.1   **1.** 7:00 P.M.   _____

9.1   **2.** 2:00 A.M.   _____

9.1   **3.** 4:00 P.M.   _____

MEDICATION RECORD | NOTE:

ADMINISTRATION PERIOD			
NO	MEDICATION DOSE, FREQUENCY	START DATE	STOP DATE
PRN 2	-MEPERIDINE 50MG/1ML AMP 50 MG Q4H PRN PAIN PRN IM	05/20/90	
		RENEW 05/24/90	
PRN 3	-DALMAME (FLURAZEPAM) 15 MG CAP 1 CAP HS PRN SLEEP PRN PO	05/20/90	
		RENEW	
PRN 4	PHENERGAN (PROMETHAZINE) 50 MG INJ 1 ML AMPULE PRN INJ	05/20/90	
		RENEW	
SCH 10	LANOXIN (DIGOXIN) 0.125 MG TAB– 1 TAB QD1300 PO CHECK PULSE	05/20/90	
		RENEW	

Figure 9–11. Medication administration record

Convert the twenty-four-hour clock time to traditional time.

9.1 **4.** 2000 _____

9.1 **5.** 1400 _____

9.1 **6.** 0900 _____

Use the MAR illustrated in Figure 9–11 to answer questions 7 through 15.

9.2 **7.** What is the generic name for Lanoxin?

_____

9.2 **8.** How often can meperidine be administered to the patient?

_____

9.2 **9.** When should Dalmane be administered?

_____

9.2 **10.** How is meperidine supplied by the pharmacy?

_____

9.2 **11.** What is the prescription number for Dalmane?

_____

9.2 **12.** Which medication is a scheduled medication?

_____

9.4. Chapter 9 Self Test

9.2 **13.** What is the generic name for Dalmane?

9.2 **14.** What is the prescription number for Lanoxin?

9.2 **15.** What are the specific instructions listed for the administration of Lanoxin?

10
Calculations for the Preparation of Solutions (Optional)

OBJECTIVES

After studying this chapter you should be able to

1. interpret solution labels;
2. calculate amounts of pure drug, solvent, or finished solution;
3. calculate the strength of solution;
4. prepare a weak solution from a strong solution.

INTRODUCTION

Most hospital pharmacies have stock supplies of the most common solutions, which are ready and available upon request. However, there may be times, especially in smaller hospitals or in rural areas, when you must assume the responsibility of preparing solutions of different strengths. In particular, you may be asked to prepare solutions for soaks, irrigations, or disinfectants.

10.1 INTERPRETING SOLUTION LABELS

A **solution** is a liquid preparation that contains a dissolved drug. It consists of a **solvent**, the liquid in which the drug is dissolved, and a **solute**, the drug added

10.1. Interpreting Solution Labels

to the solvent. When expressing solution strength, the numerator is the solute, and the denominator is the amount of finished solution.

$$\text{Solution strength} = \frac{\text{Part drug (solute)}}{\text{Amount of finished solution}}$$

Solid solutes dissolved in a solvent are usually indicated on the solution labels by the symbol **W/V** (read "weight per volume"). In a W/V solution, the solution strength must be interpreted as g/mL in the metric system or as a gr/℥ in the apothecaries' system.

Liquid solutes dissolved in a solvent are usually indicated on the solution labels by the symbol **V/V** (read "volume per volume"). In a V/V solution, the solution strength may be interpreted using any label, as long as the unit in the numerator matches the unit label in the denominator, such as oz/oz or ʒ/ʒ.

Strengths of solutions are indicated in three ways:

(a) percentage strength (25% magnesium sulfate)
(b) unlabeled ratio (isopropyl alcohol 1:2)
(c) labeled ratio (sodium bicarbonate 850 mg/5 mL)

Percentage Strength

Percentage strength is interpreted in a special way. It is the number of parts of pure drug per 100 parts of finished solution.

$$\text{\% Solution strength} = \frac{\text{Part drug}}{100 \text{ parts finished solution}}$$

EXAMPLE 10.1

Interpret the label, Magnesium sulfate 25% (W/V).

A W/V solution is interpreted as either $\frac{g}{mL}$ or $\frac{gr}{℥}$.

Metric system

$\frac{25 \text{ g}}{100 \text{ mL}}$ ← Part drug (magnesium sulfate)
← 100 parts finished solution

Apothecaries' system

$\frac{25 \text{ gr}}{100 \text{ ℥}}$ ← Part drug (magnesium sulfate)
← 100 parts finished solution

The 25% W/V magnesium sulfate solution is prepared by taking 25 g magnesium sulfate (or 25 gr) and adding enough sterile solvent to make exactly 100 mL of solution (or 100 ℥).

EXAMPLE 10.2

Interpret the label, 2% (V/V) Burow's solution.

Metric system

$$\frac{2 \text{ mL}}{100 \text{ mL}} \quad \begin{matrix}\leftarrow \text{Part drug (Burow's solution)} \\ \leftarrow \text{100 parts finished solution}\end{matrix}$$

Apothecaries' system

$$\frac{2 \text{ drams}}{100 \text{ drams}} \quad \begin{matrix}\leftarrow \text{Part drug (Burow's solution)} \\ \leftarrow \text{100 parts finished solution}\end{matrix}$$

Unlabeled Ratio

In an **unlabeled ratio,** the numerator and the denominator are interpreted as follows:

$$\text{Solution strength} = \frac{\text{Part drug}}{\text{Amount finished solution}}$$

EXAMPLE 10.3

Interpret the label, Sodium chloride 1:25 (W/V)

Metric system

$$\frac{1 \text{ g}}{25 \text{ mL}} \quad \begin{matrix}\leftarrow \text{Part drug (sodium chloride)} \\ \leftarrow \text{Amount finished solution}\end{matrix}$$

Apothecaries' system

$$\frac{1 \text{ gr}}{25 \text{ ℥}} \quad \begin{matrix}\leftarrow \text{Part drug (sodium chloride)} \\ \leftarrow \text{Amount finished solution}\end{matrix}$$

EXAMPLE 10.4

Interpret the label, Isopropyl alcohol 1:2 (V/V)

Metric system

$$\frac{1 \text{ mL}}{2 \text{ mL}} \quad \begin{matrix}\leftarrow \text{Part drug (isopropyl alcohol)} \\ \leftarrow \text{Amount finished solution}\end{matrix}$$

10.1. Interpreting Solution Labels

Apothecaries' system

$$\frac{1 \text{ oz}}{2 \text{ oz}} \begin{array}{l} \leftarrow \text{Part drug (isopropyl alcohol)} \\ \leftarrow \text{Amount finished solution} \end{array}$$

Any metric or apothecaries' unit can be used for a V/V ratio as long as the unit label is the same in both the numerator and the denominator.

EXAMPLE 10.5

Interpret the label, Silver nitrate 1:20 000 (W/V)

Metric system

$$\frac{1 \text{ g}}{20\ 000 \text{ mL}} \begin{array}{l} \leftarrow \text{Part drug (silver nitrate)} \\ \leftarrow \text{Amount finished solution} \end{array}$$

Apothecaries' system

$$\frac{1 \text{ gr}}{20\ 000 \text{ 𝔐}} \begin{array}{l} \leftarrow \text{Part drug (silver nitrate)} \\ \leftarrow \text{Amount finished solution} \end{array}$$

Labeled Ratio

In a **labeled ratio**, the label is interpreted exactly as written.

EXAMPLE 10.6

Interpret the label, Sodium bicarbonate 850 mg/5 mL. The label states exactly what the solution contains.

$$\frac{850 \text{ mg}}{5 \text{ mL}} \begin{array}{l} \leftarrow \text{Part drug (sodium bicarbonate)} \\ \leftarrow \text{Amount finished solution} \end{array}$$

PRACTICE SET 10.1

Interpret each of the following labels in both metric and apothecaries' units.

1. Epinephrine 1:20 000 (W/V)
2. Isopropyl alcohol 60% (V/V)
3. Tyloxapol 1:1000 (V/V)
4. Oxethazine 0.3% (W/V)
5. Magnesium sulfate 10% (W/V)

6. Potassium permanganate 1:20 (W/V)
7. Burow's solution 1:10 (V/V)
8. Glycerin 50% (V/V)
9. Acetaminophen elixir 150 mg/5 mL. What does this label mean?
10. A spirit of camphor solution is made by mixing 0.6 g camphor with 30 mL alcohol. Write the labeled ratio.

10.2 CALCULATING THE AMOUNT OF PURE DRUG, SOLVENT, AND FINISHED SOLUTION

The amount of drug in a solution is the quantity of the pure liquid or solid drug that is needed to make a solution of a certain strength. The amount of solvent in a solution is the amount of diluent added to the solute in order to make the required volume of finished solution. The amount of finished solution is the final volume of the solution as ordered by a physician that will contain the prescribed amount of pure drug.

The following proportion shows the relationship between the solution strength and the desired solution.

$$\underset{\downarrow}{\text{Solution strength}} \qquad \underset{\downarrow}{\text{Desired solution}}$$

$$\frac{\text{Part drug (solute)}}{\text{Amount of total solution}} = \frac{\text{Amount of drug desired (solute)}}{\text{Amount of finished solution desired}}$$

Rule 10.1 gives the steps for calculating the amount of pure drug or finished solution.

RULE 10.1 Rule for Calculating the Amount of Pure Drug or the Finished Solution

Step 1. Write the solution strength as a ratio.

$$\text{Solution strength} = \frac{\text{Part drug (solute)}}{\text{Amount of total solution}}$$

Step 2. Write the desired solution as a ratio.

$$\text{Desired solution} = \frac{\text{Amount of drug desired}}{\text{Amount of finished solution desired}}$$

Step 3. Set ratios equal to each other and solve for x.

10.2. Calculating the Amount of Pure Drug, Solvent, and Finished Solution

EXAMPLE 10.7

A doctor prescribes 7.5 mL of Feosol elixir for a patient. The solution label reads 220 mg/5 mL. How many mg of the pure drug did the patient receive?

Step 1. → $\underset{\text{Solution strength}}{\dfrac{220 \text{ mg}}{5 \text{ mL}}} = \underset{\text{Desired strength}}{\dfrac{x \text{ mg}}{7.5 \text{ mL}}}$ ← Step 2.

Step 3.
$$5x = (220)(7.5)$$
$$5x = 1650$$
$$x = 330 \text{ mg}$$

Answer. The patient received 330 mg of Feosol.

EXAMPLE 10.8

A doctor prescribes 200 000 mcg Methocarbamol for an intramuscular (IM) injection. Methocarbamol 1:10 (W/V) solution is available. How many mL will you administer?

Since this is an unlabeled ratio (W/V) and since mL are asked for, use the metric interpretation $\left(\dfrac{g}{mL}\right)$ for the label.

Interpret 1:10 (W/V) as 1 g/10 mL

$$\textit{Part drug} = 1 \text{ g}$$
$$\textit{Amount of total solution} = 10 \text{ mL}$$
$$\textit{Amount of drug desired} = 200\,000 \text{ mcg}$$
$$\textit{Amount of finished solution} = x \text{ mL}$$

Substitute these amounts in the proportion,

$$\text{Solution strength} = \text{Desired solution}$$

Steps 1–2.   1:10 (W/V) → $\underset{\text{Solution strength}}{\dfrac{1 \text{ g}}{10 \text{ mL}}} = \underset{\text{Desired solution}}{\dfrac{200\,000 \text{ mcg}}{x \text{ mL}}}$

Changing to like unit labels in the numerators,

$$200\,000 \text{ mcg} = 0.2 \text{ g}$$

By substitution:

Step 3. $\dfrac{1 \text{ g}}{10 \text{ mL}} = \dfrac{0.2 \text{ g}}{x \text{ mL}} \quad \leftarrow 200\,000 \text{ mcg}$

$$1x = (0.2)(10)$$
$$x = 2 \text{ mL}$$

Answer. Administer 2 mL of 1:10 (W/V) Methocarbamol.

Rule 10.2 can be used as a guide when writing preparations. This rule should be used along with this proportion:

$$\frac{\text{Part drug}}{\text{Amount of total solution}} = \frac{\text{Amount of drug desired}}{\text{Amount of finished solution desired}}$$

RULE 10.2   Rule for Writing a Preparation

Fill the parentheses with the appropriate amounts. Take (*numerator of right ratio*) of (*drug*) and add enough sterile solvent to make exactly (*denominator of right ratio*).

EXAMPLE 10.9

A doctor orders sterile warm 5% (W/V) boric acid compresses for a patient. In order to prepare 1 000 mL of boric acid solution, how many grams of boric acid crystals should be used? Write the preparation for this solution.

Interpret 5% (W/V) as 5 g/100 mL

$$\text{Part drug} = 5 \text{ g}$$
$$\text{Amount of total solution} = 100 \text{ mL}$$
$$\text{Amount of drug desired} = x \text{ g}$$
$$\text{Amount of finished solution} = 1000 \text{ mL}$$

10.2. Calculating the Amount of Pure Drug, Solvent, and Finished Solution

$$5\% \rightarrow \underset{\text{Solution strength}}{\frac{5 \text{ g}}{100 \text{ mL}}} = \underset{\text{Desired solution}}{\frac{x \text{ g}}{1000 \text{ mL}}}$$

$$100x = (5)(1000)$$
$$100x = 5000$$
$$x = 50 \text{ g}$$

Use Rule 10.2 to write the preparation.

Preparation: Take *50 g* (numerator) of *boric acid crystals* (drug) and add enough sterile solvent to make exactly *1000 mL* (denominator).

EXAMPLE 10.10

Prepare 200 mL of 10% (V/V) glycerin solution. Write the preparation.

$$10\% \rightarrow \underset{\text{Solution strength}}{\frac{10 \text{ mL}}{100 \text{ mL}}} = \underset{\text{Desired solution}}{\frac{x \text{ mL}}{200 \text{ mL}}}$$

$$100x = (10)(200)$$
$$x = 20 \text{ mL}$$

Use Rule 10.2 to write the preparation.

Preparation: Take *20 mL* of *glycerin* and add enough sterile solvent to make exactly *200 mL*.

PRACTICE SET 10.2

1. A 200 cc solution of 20% (W/V) boric acid is needed for compresses. How many g of boric acid crystals are needed to prepare this 20% solution?

2. A 1:50 (W/V) solution of sodium perborate is needed for a mouthwash. How many mL of mouthwash can be made from 2 g of sodium perborate? Write the preparation.

3. How many cc of a 10% (W/V) solution can be made from 10 g of a drug?

212   10.   Calculations for the Preparation of Solutions (Optional)

4. Prepare 150 mL of 0.02% (W/V) Ceepryn chloride for application to wounds.

5. Dr. Zemer ordered 110 mL of a 0.9% (W/V) saline gargle for a patient suffering from a sore throat. How many g of sodium chloride are needed to make this solution? Write the preparation.

6. Prepare 200 mL of a 1:100 (V/V) vinegar solution to be used as a vaginal douche.

7. Order: Magnesium sulfate 5.5% (W/V); 250 mL for a soak. Available: Magnesium sulfate (Epsom salts). Write the preparation.

8. Dr. Sun ordered 9.5 mL of Feosol elixir for a patient. The solution label reads 220 mg/50 mL. How many mg did the patient receive?

9. Order: 250 000 mcg Methocarbamol IM. Available: 10% (W/V) Methocarbamol. How many mL will you administer?

10. Prepare 1 L of a 1:20 000 (W/V) silver nitrate solution for a bladder irrigation.

EXAMPLE 10.11

Administer gr $\frac{1}{250}$ of 0.05 (W/V) solution of a drug. How many ℳ will you give?

Since this is a (W/V) solution, and since the answer calls for ℳ, use the apothecaries' interpretation of the label 0.05%.

$$0.05\% \rightarrow \frac{0.05 \text{ gr}}{100 \text{ ℳ}} = \frac{\frac{1}{250} \text{ gr}}{x \text{ ℳ}}$$

(Solution strength → ; Desired solution ↓)

Since $\frac{1}{250} = 0.004$, by substitution:

$$\frac{0.05 \text{ gr}}{100 \text{ ℳ}} = \frac{0.004 \text{ gr}}{x \text{ ℳ}}$$

$$0.05x = (0.004)(100)$$

$$x = 8$$

Answer.   Administer 8ℳ of the 0.05% (W/V) solution.

EXAMPLE 10.12

Prepare 60 mL of 1:10 (W/V) sodium bicarbonate solution. If sodium bicarbonate gr x tablets are available, how many tabs will you use?

Divide the problem into two parts. In Part 1, find the amount of drug needed

10.2. Calculating the Amount of Pure Drug, Solvent, and Finished Solution 213

for the solution. In Part 2, find the number of tabs that will be needed to make the exact amount of pure drug.

Part 1. Find the amount of pure drug needed for the 1:10 (W/V) solution. Use the metric interpretation for the label.

$$1{:}10\ (W/V) \rightarrow \frac{\overset{\text{Solution strength}}{\downarrow}}{\underset{10\ \text{mL}}{1\ \text{g}}} = \frac{\overset{\text{Desired solution}}{\downarrow}}{\underset{60\ \text{mL}}{x\ \text{g}}}$$

$$10x = 60$$

$$x = 6\ \text{g}$$

Part 2. Find the number of gr x tablets needed to make 6 g of pure drug.

$$\frac{\overset{\text{MOH}}{\downarrow}}{\underset{1\ \text{tab}}{10\ \text{gr}}} = \frac{\overset{\text{DM}}{\downarrow}}{\underset{x\ \text{tabs}}{6\ \text{g}}}$$

Change 6 g to gr (using 1 g = 15 gr) and substitute.

$$\frac{\overset{\text{MOH}}{\downarrow}}{\underset{1\ \text{tab}}{10\ \text{gr}}} = \frac{\overset{\text{DM}}{\downarrow}}{\underset{x\ \text{tabs}}{90\ \text{gr}}}$$

$$x = 9$$

Answer. Use 9 tabs of sodium bicarbonate (gr x/tab) to make the 1:10 (W/V) solution of sodium bicarbonate.

EXAMPLE 10.13

Prepare 1 qt of 1:5 (V/V) hydrogen peroxide.

$$1{:}5\ (V/V) \rightarrow \frac{\overset{\text{Solution strength}}{\downarrow}}{\underset{5\ \text{qt}}{1\ \text{qt}}} = \frac{\overset{\text{Desired solution}}{\downarrow}}{\underset{1\ \text{qt}}{x\ \text{qt}}}$$

$$5x = 1$$

$$x = \frac{1}{5}\ \text{qt}$$

Preparation: Take $\frac{1}{5}$ qt of hydrogen peroxide and add enough sterile solvent to make exactly 1 qt.

There is a difference in the amount of solvent needed when working with a W/V or a V/V solution. For example, when sodium chloride is added to sterile water in a W/V solution, the salt dissolves, but more important, the total volume of water does not appreciably increase. On the other hand, when preparing a V/V solution, such as 50 mL of hydrogen peroxide mixed with 100 mL of sterile water, the amount of finished solution is 150 mL—a marked difference in total volume. Thus, in making a V/V solution, measure the solute first and then add just enough solvent to make the required finished solution. Rule 10.3 states how to calculate the amount of solvent to be added in a V/V solution.

RULE 10.3 Rule for Calculating Amount of Solvent in a V/V Solution

Amount of solvent = Amount of finished solution − Amount of solute

---

EXAMPLE 10.14

How many mL of sterile water should you add to 45 mL of glycerol to make a 0.5% (V/V) solution?

Divide the problem into two parts.

Part 1. Find the amount of finished solution.

$$0.5\% \rightarrow \frac{0.5 \text{ mL}}{100 \text{ mL}} = \frac{45 \text{ mL}}{x \text{ mL}}$$

(Solution strength ↓ ; Desired solution ↓)

$$0.5x = (45)(100)$$
$$x = 9000 \text{ mL}$$

The amount of finished solution is 9000 mL.

Part 2. Find the amount of solvent (water) to be added to the 45 mL of pure drug to make 9000 mL of finished solution. Use Rule 10.3.

Amount of solvent = Amount of finished solution − Amount of solute

Amount of solvent = 9000 mL − 45 mL

Amount of solvent = 8955 mL

Answer. Add 8 955 mL of sterile water to the 45 mL glycerol to make 9000 mL of 0.5% (V/V) glycerol solution.

EXAMPLE 10.15

A glycerin solution 25% (V/V) is available. An order calls for glycerin 1.5 mL/kg body mass. How many mL will you administer to a 143-lb patient?

Divide the problem into three parts.

Part 1. Convert 143 lb. to kg.

$$\frac{2.2 \text{ lb}}{1 \text{ kg}} = \frac{143 \text{ lb}}{x \text{ kg}}$$

$$2.2x = (1)(143)$$

$$x = 65 \text{ kg}$$

Part 2. Calculate the drug dosage for the 65-kg patient.

$$\frac{1.5 \text{ mL}}{1 \text{ kg}} = \frac{x \text{ mL}}{65 \text{ kg}}$$

$$1x = (1.5)(65)$$

$$x = 97.5 \text{ mL of pure glycerin}$$

Part 3. Calculate amount of desired solution.

$$25\% \rightarrow \frac{25 \text{ mL}}{100 \text{ mL}} = \frac{97.5 \text{ mL}}{x \text{ mL}}$$

(Solution strength ↓   Desired solution ↓)

$$25x = (100)(97.5)$$

$$25x = 9750$$

$$x = 390 \text{ mL}$$

Answer. Administer 390 mL of the 25% (V/V) glycerin solution to the patient.

PRACTICE SET 10.2 (cont.)

11. How many L of 1:10 (V/V) Burow's solution can be made from 250 mL concentrated Burow's solution?

12. 500 mL of 1:20 (W/V) solution glucose is desired. How many g of crystalline glucose are needed? Write the preparation for the 1:20 (W/V) solution of glucose.

13. How much sodium bicarbonate is needed to make 300 mL of 10% (W/V) sodium bicarbonate solution? Write the preparation.

14. Prepare 200 mL of 1:50 (V/V) silver nitrate solution.

15. How many ᷓ of 8% (V/V) Burow's solution can be made from 500 ᷓ of concentrated Burow's solution?

16. How many mL of sterile solvent must be added to 50 mL of glycerin in order to make a 25% (V/V) solution?

17. An order calls for Mercurochrome 0.275 g. Mercurochrome 15 mg/mL is available. How many mL will you administer?

18. A 50 cc vial contains 5.5% (W/V) sodium bicarbonate solution. How many mg of sodium bicarbonate are in the vial?

19. 1000 mL of 0.35% (W/V) sodium chloride and 3.5% (W/V) dextrose solution will contain how many g sodium chloride and how many g dextrose?

20. A patient weighs 88 lb. A physician prescribes a 25% (W/V) mannitol solution 1.5 g/kg body mass. How many mL should the patient receive?

10.3 CALCULATING THE STRENGTH OF A SOLUTION

Sometimes you will have to calculate the strength of a solution and label the stock bottle once the solution is made. Rule 10.4 will help you calculate the percentage strength.

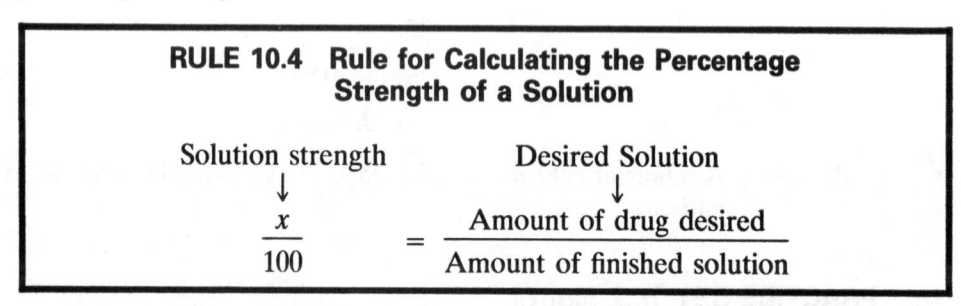

RULE 10.4 Rule for Calculating the Percentage Strength of a Solution

Solution strength → $\dfrac{x}{100}$ = $\dfrac{\text{Amount of drug desired}}{\text{Amount of finished solution}}$ ← Desired Solution

---

When using this proportion to calculate the percentage strength of a solution, the denominator of the solution strength is always 100, since percentage means parts per 100. The only units that can be used in this proportion for a W/V solution are g/mL or gr/℥. Any unit can be used for a V/V solution.

10.3. Calculating the Strength of a Solution

EXAMPLE 10.16

50 gr of sodium bromide have been dissolved in 150 ℳ of sterile solvent. What is the % sodium bromide solution?

$$\text{Meaning of \%} \rightarrow \underset{\text{Solution strength}}{\frac{x \text{ gr}}{100}} = \underset{\text{Desired strength}}{\frac{50 \text{ gr}}{150 \text{ ℳ}}}$$

$$150x = (50)(100)$$
$$150x = 5000$$
$$x = 33\frac{1}{3}$$

$$\text{Solution strength} = \frac{33\frac{1}{3}}{100} = 33\frac{1}{3}\%$$

Answer. 50 gr of sodium bromide dissolved in 150 ℳ of sterile solvent constitutes a $33\frac{1}{3}\%$ sodium bromide solution.

EXAMPLE 10.17

What is the percentage strength of 300 000 mcg dissolved in 10 mL solution?

$$\text{Meaning of \%} \rightarrow \underset{\text{Solution strength}}{\frac{x \text{ g}}{100 \text{ mL}}} = \underset{\text{Desired solution}}{\frac{300\,000 \text{ mcg}}{10 \text{ mL}}}$$

By substitution, 300 000 mcg = 0.3 g. (For %, the solution strength must be interpreted g/mL or gr/ℳ.)

$$\frac{x \text{ g}}{100 \text{ mL}} = \frac{0.3 \text{ g}}{10 \text{ mL}}$$
$$10x = (0.3)(100)$$
$$x = 3$$

$$\text{Solution strength} = \frac{3 \text{ g}}{100 \text{ mL}} = 3\%$$

Answer. The percentage strength of 300 000 mcg dissolved in 10 mL solution is 3%.

To calculate the unlabeled ratio for a solution, find the percentage strength first and then reduce this percentage ratio to lowest terms. The reduced ratio is the unlabeled ratio.

EXAMPLE 10.18

A solution has been prepared by dissolving 500 mg of iodine crystals in 10 mL of solution. Write the solution strength as an unlabeled ratio.

Divide the problem into two parts. In Part 1, find the percentage strength. In Part 2, reduce the percentage strength ratio to lowest terms. This will be the unlabeled ratio.

Part 1.

Meaning of % → $\dfrac{x \text{ g}}{100 \text{ mL}} = \dfrac{0.5 \text{ g}}{10 \text{ mL}}$ ← 500 mg

(Solution strength ↓ ; Desired solution ↓)

$$10x = (100)(0.5)$$
$$10x = 50$$
$$x = 5$$

Solution strength = $\dfrac{5}{100}$

Part 2. Take the percentage solution strength ratio and reduce it to lowest terms.

$$\dfrac{5}{100} = \dfrac{1}{20}$$

Unlabeled ratio = 1:20

Answer. 500 mg of iodine crystals dissolved in 10 mL of solution is a 1:20 (W/V) iodine solution.

EXAMPLE 10.19

What is the unlabeled ratio strength of 1 qt of Lysol solution containing 200 mL of pure Lysol?

Part 1. Find the percentage strength.

10.3. Calculating the Strength of a Solution

Meaning of % → $\dfrac{x \text{ mL}}{100 \text{ mL}}$ = $\dfrac{200 \text{ mL}}{1000 \text{ mL}}$ ← 1 qt changed to mL

$$1000x = (100)(200)$$
$$1000x = 20\,000$$
$$x = 20$$

Solution strength = $\dfrac{20}{100}$

Part 2. Reduce the percentage strength to lowest terms to find the unlabeled ratio.

$$\dfrac{20}{100} = \dfrac{1}{5}$$

Unlabeled ratio = 1:5

Answer. 200 mL of Lysol in a 1 qt solution of Lysol is a 1:5 (V/V) solution.

For a labeled ratio, write the exact amount of drug contained in the exact amount of solution on the label.

EXAMPLE 10.20

An iodine solution 1000 mg/20 mL has been made. What is the labeled ratio?

Answer. 1000 mg/20 mL iodine solution.

PRACTICE SET 10.3

1. 15 g of iodine are dissolved in 1 L of solution. What is the percentage strength?

2. A 500 cc container of dextrose solution contains 2.5 g of pure dextrose. What is the unlabeled ratio strength?

3. A solution has been prepared by dissolving 2.25 gr in a diluent sufficient to make 150 ℳ of solution. Express the solution strength both as a percentage and as an unlabeled ratio.

4. What is the percentage strength and the unlabeled ratio of a 2 pt solution containing 40 g of sodium chloride?

5. A solution of sodium bromide has been prepared by dissolving 1 500 mg of sodium bromide in 100 mL of solution. Express the solution strength as a percent, an unlabeled ratio, and a labeled ratio.

6. 20 g of solute are dissolved in 400 cc of sterile water. Write the percentage strength.

7. A 5 mL solution contains 100 mg of a drug. What is the unlabeled ratio for this solution?

8. 20 mL of a V/V solution contains 2 mL pure drug. What is the percentage strength and the unlabeled ratio?

9. A solution of 50 g of Epsom salts per 250 mL of sterile water has been prepared for a soak. Write the unlabeled ratio and the labeled ratio for this solution.

10. Four tabs of mercuric chloride (gr viiss/tab) have been dissolved in 80 cc of sterile water. Write the percentage strength and the unlabeled ratio for this mercuric chloride solution.

10.4 PREPARING A WEAK SOLUTION FROM A STRONG SOLUTION

Concentrated solutions are available in the pharmacy or in the stock room. If a physician orders a weaker solution, these stock solutions must be diluted. Rule 10.5 can be used to prepare a weak solution from a strong solution.

RULE 10.5 Rule for Preparing a Weak Solution from a Strong Solution

$$\text{Amount of drug in strong solution} = \text{Amount of drug in weak solution}$$

$$(V_s)(S_s) = (V_w)(S_w)$$

where V_s = Volume of strong solution, S_s = Strength of strong solution, V_w = Volume of weak solution, S_w = Strength of weak solution.

The amount of drug in the strong solution does not differ from the amount of drug in the weak solution. What does differ is the amount of solvent.

EXAMPLE 10.21

How many L of a 10% Lysol solution are needed to prepare 1 L of a 3% Lysol solution?

10.4. Preparing a Weak Solution from a Strong Solution

Use Rule 10.5.

$$\begin{array}{ccc} \text{Amount of drug} & & \text{Amount of drug} \\ \text{in} & = & \text{in} \\ \text{strong solution} & & \text{weak solution} \\ \downarrow & & \downarrow \\ (V_s)(S_s) & = & (V_w)(S_w) \\ (x \text{ L})(10\%) & = & (1 \text{ L})(3\%) \\ & x = 0.3 \text{ L} & \end{array}$$

Answer. 0.3 L of a 10% Lysol solution is needed.

Rule 10.6 can be used as a model for writing the preparation of a weak solution from a strong solution.

RULE 10.6 Rule for Preparing a Weak Solution from a Strong Solution

Fill the parentheses with the appropriate amount. Take (V_s) of the $(S_s$ drug) and add enough sterile solvent to make exactly (V_w) of the $(S_w$ drug) solution.

For Example 10.21, the preparation is:

(V_s) (S_s) (drug)
↓   ↓   ↓

Take *0.3 L* of the *10% Lysol* solution and add enough sterile solvent to make exactly *1 liter* of the 3% Lysol solution.
↑   ↑
(V_w) (S_w)

EXAMPLE 10.22

Prepare 1500 mL of Zephiran Chloride 1:20 000 solution from 1:1000 Zephiran Chloride solution.

Use Rule 10.5.

$$\begin{array}{cccc} (V_s) & (S_s) & = & (V_w) & (S_w) \\ \downarrow & \downarrow & & \downarrow & \downarrow \\ (x \text{ mL})(1:1000) & = & (1500 \text{ mL}) & (1:20\,000) \end{array}$$

Change the unlabeled ratios to decimal form.

$$\begin{array}{cc} 1:1000 & 1:20\,000 \\ \downarrow & \downarrow \\ (x \text{ mL})(0.001) = (1\,500 \text{ mL})(0.00005) \\ x = 75 \text{ mL} \end{array}$$

Preparation: Take *75 mL* of the *1:1000* Zephiran Chloride and add enough sterile solvent to make exactly *1500 mL* of the *1:20 000* Zephiran Chloride solution.

EXAMPLE 10.23

How much Merthiolate 0.0025% solution can be made from 40 mL of 1:200 solution of Merthiolate?

Sometimes it is difficult to judge which is the stronger solution if one strength is written in a percentage form and the other is written in an unlabeled ratio form. If you change each strength to its decimal equivalent, you can more easily select the stronger solution.

$$1:200 = 0.005$$
$$0.0025\% = 0.000025$$

0.000025 is the weak solution, and 0.005 is the strong solution. Substitute the decimal equivalents into the rule and solve for x.

$$(V_s)(S_s) = (V_w)(S_w)$$
$$(40 \text{ mL})(1:200) = (x \text{ mL})(0.0025\%)$$
$$(40 \text{ mL})(0.005) = (x \text{ mL})(0.000025)$$
$$x = 8000 \text{ mL}$$

Answer. 8000 mL Merthiolate solution can be made from 40 mL of 1:200 Merthiolate solution.

PRACTICE SET 10.4

1. Prepare 1000 mL of 1:1000 potassium permanganate solution from a 1:10 potassium permanganate solution.

2. Prepare 500 mL of a 25% creosol solution from a 1:2 creosol solution.

3. How many mL of a 1% solution of formaldehyde can be made from 50 mL of 50% solution of formaldehyde?

4. How much sterile water needs to be added to a gal of 65% isopropyl alcohol to make it a 50% solution?

5. How much 6% sodium chloride solution is needed to make 1000 mL of 0.9% solution?

6. Prepare 500 mL of a 1:5000 solution from a 25% solution. Write the preparation.

7. Ceepryn chloride is ordered by a physician to be applied to a patient's wounds. Ceepryn chloride 0.1% is available. Prepare 200 mL of 0.02% Ceepryn chloride for the application.

8. Prepare 1000 mL of 1:100 formaldehyde solution. A 75% solution is available.

9. How much sterile solvent must be added to 200 mL of a 10% solution to make a 5% solution?

10. Cupric sulfate 1:4000 is needed as a fungicidal agent. If cupric sulfate 5% is available, how would you prepare 300 mL?

11. Order: 450 mL nitrofurazone 0.1% solution.
    Available: 0.2% nitrofurazone.
    Write the preparation.

12. Order: 800 mL 1:20 000 Zephiran Chloride solution.
    Available: 1:1000 Zephiran Chloride.
    Write the preparation.

13. A physician orders 400 mL of 1:4000 cupric sulfate for use as a fungicidal agent. How many mL 5% cupric sulfate solution are needed to make this solution?

14. How much solvent needs to be added to 250 mL of 2% Mercurochrome to make it a 1% solution?

15. How many mL of 1:20 sodium bicarbonate solution can be made from 10 mL of 1:10 sodium bicarbonate solution?

10.5 CHAPTER 10 REVIEW PROBLEMS

1. Prepare 200 mL of cupric sulfate 1:400 for use as a fungicidal agent. Cupric sulfate 5% is available.

2. You are preparing sodium perborate 1:50 (W/V) solution for a mouthwash. How many grams of sodium perborate should you use to prepare 200 mL of solution?

3. 500 mg of iodine are dissolved in 1 L of sodium iodide. What is the percentage strength?

4. Prepare a 25% (W/V) solution of sodium chloride from 200 g of sodium chloride.

5. Prepare 200 mL of a 3% acetic acid solution. Acetic acid 6% solution is available.

6. How many mL of 0.9% (W/V) silver nitrate can be made from 300 mg of silver nitrate crystals?

7. Order: 150 mcg gynergen tartrate. Available: 1:20 000 (W/V). How many mL will you administer?

8. How many mL of a 2% (W/V) solution can be made from 460 mg of codeine sulfate?

9. What is the unlabeled ratio strength of a solution in which 4 pt contain 80 g of a drug?

10. How many g of sodium carbonate are needed to prepare 0.5 L of a 6% (W/V) sodium carbonate solution?

11. Prepare 500 mL of 1:200 dextrose solution from $2\frac{1}{2}$% dextrose solution.

12. Prepare 150 mL 0.02% Ceepryn chloride for application to wounds. Ceepryn chloride 0.1% solution is available.

13. How many g of potassium permanganate are needed to prepare 250 mL of a 2% (W/V) solution?

14. 0.25 g of potassium permanganate crystals are dissolved in 500 mL of finished solution. What is the percentage strength and the unlabeled ratio for this potassium permanganate solution?

15. How many mL of stock solution of 50% alcohol would you use to prepare 2 L of 25% alcohol solution?

16. How many g of iodine crystals would be needed to prepare ℥ iv of 10% (W/V) iodine solution?

17. How many mL of a 25% stock solution of formaldehyde is needed to prepare 1 L of a 2% solution?

18. How many ℥ of 5% (V/V) glucose solution can be made from ℥ xxiiss of glucose solute?

19. A 50 cc vial contains 150 mg of sodium bromide. What is the % sodium bromide solution in this vial?

20. How much sterile water needs to be added to 0.5 L of 75% isopropyl alcohol to change it to a 30% solution?

21. Administer gr $\frac{1}{100}$ of a drug. 0.04% (W/V) solution is available. How many ℳ will you administer?

10.5. Chapter 10 Review Problems

22. What is the percentage strength of ℨ v silver nitrate solution containing 15 g silver nitrate?

23. How much Argyrol 3% solution can be prepared from 150 mL Argyrol 5% solution?

24. Potassium iodide 75% (W/V) is available in a 50 cc vial. Administer 375 mg of potassium iodide. How many *drops* will you administer?

25. An oral suspension of oxethazaine 0.3% (W/V) is available. If an order calls for 10 000 mcg, how many mL will you administer?

26. A doctor prescribes salicylate gr xx for a patient. The medication on hand is a 16% (W/V) solution. How many gtt (𝔐) will you administer?

27. Prepare 5 gal of 1:5000 (W/V) solution of mercuric chloride from gr viiss tablets.

28. How many 𝔐 of a 1:1000 (W/V) solution can be made from 2 tabs of gr $\frac{1}{4}$ drug?

29. A physician prescribes magnesium sulfate 100 mg/kg body mass for a 110-lb patient in two equally divided doses. Magnesium sulfate 75% (W/V) solution is available. How much will you administer per dose?

30. A doctor orders epinephrine 10 mg/kg body mass in two equally divided doses for a 90-lb patient. Epinephrine 1:500 (W/V) is available. How much will you administer per dose?

31. A solution has been prepared by dissolving 2.25 gr in diluent sufficient to make 10 mL of solution. Express the solution strength as a percentage and as an unlabeled ratio.

32. Prepare a 20% (W/V) solution of sodium bicarbonate from 125 g of the drug.

33. A 500 cc container of a dextrose solution contains 2.5 g of pure dextrose. What is the unlabeled ratio strength?

34. How many ℨ water would you add to ℨ iss of glycerol to make a 0.5% (V/V) solution?

35. How much 4% Lysol solution can be made from 5 L of 1:20 solution?

36. 15 g of iodine are dissolved in 1 L of sodium iodide. What is the percentage strength?

37. A 60-lb child is to receive medication 8 mg/kg body mass. The medication available is 160 mg/12 mL. How many mL should the patient receive?

38. A physician prescribes magnesium sulfate 150 mg/kg body mass. Magnesium sulfate 25% (W/V) is available. If the patient's mass is 110 lb, how many mL will you administer?

39. Administer gr $\frac{1}{200}$ using a 0.05% (W/V) solution. How many ℳ will you administer?

40. Merthiolate 0.003% is needed for a urethral irrigation. 9 mL of 1% Merthiolate solution is available in the stock room. How many L 0.003% Merthiolate solution can be prepared from the 9 mL?

41. Prepare 25 mL of a 1% (W/V) gentian violet solution. Use rubbing alcohol as the solvent.

42. Dr. Chang ordered 300 mL of a 0.5% (W/V) hydrocortisone solution to be used as a lotion for a rash. Prepare the solution using a lotion as the solvent.

43. A 25% (V/V) glycerin solution is needed. How many oz of sterile water should be added to $10\frac{1}{2}$ oz of pure glycerin to make this 25% solution?

44. Six tabs of mercuric chloride (0.5 g/tab) have been dissolved in 150 cc of sterile water. Write the percentage strength and the unlabeled ratio for this solution.

45. Order: 0.5 L of 1:5 (W/V) potassium permanganate solution. Available: potassium permanganate crystals. Write the preparation.

10.6 CHAPTER 10 SELF TEST

10.2   **1.** If a patient receives ℳ cc of an atropine sulfate 1:10 (W/V) solution, how many gr does he receive? _____

10.4   **2.** Prepare 2 L of 1:200 saponated solution of creosol from a 1:50 solution. Preparation: _____
_____

10.2   **3.** How many mL of a 0.15% (W/V) solution can be made from 0.5 g of a drug? _____

10.6. Chapter 10 Self Test

10.3   **4.** A solution has been prepared by dissolving gr $\frac{1}{8}$ in ℨ CXXV solution.

What is the percentage solution strength?

10.2   **5.** Prepare 250 mL of a 3% (W/V) boric acid solution from boric acid crystals. Preparation: _____

10.4   **6.** Prepare a 1% solution from 1 L of a 1:50 strength solution. Preparation: _____

10.2   **7.** An order calls for 30 mg codeine. The vial contains gr $\overline{ss}$/mL. How many mL should you administer?

10.2   **8.** A doctor orders 40 g glucose to be given intravenously (IV). How many mL 5% (W/V) glucose solution should be administered?

10.3   **9.** How many mL of sterile water need to be *added to* a mL of 1% Merthiolate solution to change it to a 0.002% solution?

10.2   **10.** Glycerin solution 25% (V/V) is available. A physician prescribes glycerin 1.5 mL/kg body mass for a 44-lb patient. How many mL of the 25% (V/V) solution will you administer?

10.2   **11.** Order: 115 mL of 5% (W/V) magnesium sulfate solution for a soak solution. How many grams of magnesium sulfate crystals should be used?

10.3   **12.** 5 grams of potassium permanganate are placed in a 500 mL graduate. It is filled with distilled water up to the 500 mL mark. What is the unlabeled ratio for this potassium permanganate solution?

10.2   **13.** The doctor prescribes 0.05 mg epinephrine for a patient's asthma. A 1:10 000 (W/V) solution is available. How much should be administered to the patient?

10.2 **14.** 300 mL of sodium chloride 5% (W/V) have been administered to a patient over the last five hours. How many g of sodium chloride has the patient received?

10.3 **15.** 0.5 gram of camphor has been mixed with alcohol to make a 50 mL spirit of camphor solution. What is the percentage strength of the solution?

SUMMARY OF CHAPTER 10 RULES

RULE 10.1 Rule for Calculating the Amount of Pure Drug or the Finished Solution

Step 1. Write the solution strength as a ratio.

$$\text{Solution strength} = \frac{\text{Part drug (solute)}}{\text{Amount of total solution}}$$

Step 2. Write the desired solution as a ratio.

$$\text{Desired solution} = \frac{\text{Amount of drug desired}}{\text{Amount of finished solution desired}}$$

Step 3. Set ratios equal to each other and solve for x.

RULE 10.2 Rule for Writing a Preparation

Fill the parentheses with the appropriate amounts. Take (*numerator of right ratio*) of (*drug*) and add enough sterile solvent to make exactly (*denominator of right ratio*).

RULE 10.3 Rule for Calculating Amount of Solvent in a V/V Solution

Amount of solvent = Amount of finished solution − Amount of solute

---

RULE 10.4 Rule for Calculating the Percentage Strength of a Solution

$$\underset{\downarrow}{\text{Solution strength}} \qquad \underset{\downarrow}{\text{Desired solution}}$$

$$\frac{x}{100} = \frac{\text{Amount of drug desired}}{\text{Amount of finished solution}}$$

RULE 10.5 Rule for Preparing a Weak Solution from a Strong Solution

$$\underset{\downarrow}{\begin{array}{c}\text{Amount of drug}\\ \text{in}\\ \text{strong solution}\end{array}} = \underset{\downarrow}{\begin{array}{c}\text{Amount of drug}\\ \text{in}\\ \text{weak solution}\end{array}}$$

$$\begin{pmatrix}\text{Volume of}\\ \text{strong}\\ \text{solution}\end{pmatrix} \begin{pmatrix}\text{Strength of}\\ \text{strong}\\ \text{solution}\end{pmatrix} = \begin{pmatrix}\text{Volume of}\\ \text{weak}\\ \text{solution}\end{pmatrix} \begin{pmatrix}\text{Strength of}\\ \text{weak}\\ \text{solution}\end{pmatrix}$$

$$(V_s) \qquad (S_s) \qquad = \qquad (V_w) \qquad (S_w)$$

RULE 10.6 Rule for Preparing a Weak Solution from a Strong Solution

Fill the parentheses with the appropriate amount. Take (V_s) of the $(S_s$ drug) and add enough sterile solvent to make exactly (V_w) of the $(S_w$ drug) solution.

APPENDIX I
Roman Numerals

Traditionally, Roman numerals are expressed using capital letters of the alphabet. In the medical field, however, lower case letters are used. Table A–1 shows the Roman numerals and their Arabic equivalents.

TABLE A–1 ROMAN NUMERALS AND THEIR EQUIVALENTS

Traditional Roman numerals	Apothecaries' Roman numerals	Arabic equivalents
I	i	1
V	v	5
X	x	10
L	l	50
C	c	100
D	d	500
M	m	1000

There are four common rules for expressing numbers in the Roman system.

RULE A.1 Succession Rule

When Roman numerals are repeated in succession, add them. The same symbol must never be repeated more than three times in succession. (Never repeat v, l, or d because when doubled, their values equal x, c, and m, respectively.)

Appendix I. Roman Numerals

EXAMPLE A.1

(a) cc = 100 + 100 = 200

(b) 22 = 10 + 10 + 1 + 1 = xxii

RULE A.2 Addition Rule

When a Roman numeral is *followed by* a lesser-valued numeral, the values are *added* together to obtain the total value.

EXAMPLE A.2

(a) xvi = 10 + 5 + 1 = 16

(b) 56 = 50 + 5 + 1 = lvi

RULE A.3 Subtraction Rule

When a lesser-valued numeral *precedes* a greater-valued numeral, the lesser-valued numeral is *subtracted* from the greater-valued numeral to obtain the total value.

EXAMPLE A.3

(a) iv = 5 − 1 = 4

(b) 40 = 50 − 10 = xl

There are a few exceptions to this rule. They are:

$$49 = \text{xlix, } not \text{ il}$$
$$99 = \text{xcix, } not \text{ ic}$$
$$490 = \text{cdxc, } not \text{ xd}$$
$$990 = \text{cmxc, } not \text{ xm}$$

RULE A.4 In-Between Rule

When a lesser-valued numeral appears *between* two greater-valued numerals, the subtraction rule takes precedence. The difference is then added to the value of the other numerals.

EXAMPLE A.4

mcd = _____

              mcd   ← The c is between two greater-valued numerals. Thus the subtraction rule takes precedence.

      m   cd
      ↓   ↓
  1000 (500 − 100)

  1000 + (500 − 100)

  1000 + 400 = 1400

Thus mcd = 1400

EXAMPLE A.5

ccxliv = _____

          ccxliv   ← The x is between two greater-valued numerals, and i is also between two greater-valued numerals

  cc   xl   iv
  ↓   ↓   ↓
  200 (50 − 10)(5 − 1)

  200 + (50 − 10) + (5 − 1) =

  200 + 40 + 4 = 244

Thus ccxliv = 244

PRACTICE SET A.1

Write the Arabic equivalent of the following:

1. cdxl
2. lxix
3. mmcccxxxii
4. dcclxxiv
5. xcviii
6. xxiiss̄
7. cdxix
8. cmlix
9. xxxiii
10. xliv
11. lxiv
12. xcviii
13. lxxxix
14. xvi
15. xiv

Write the apothecaries' Roman numeral equivalent of the following:

16. 349
17. 906
18. 51
19. 1499
20. $88\frac{1}{2}$

Practice Set A.1 Answers

21. 55	22. 29	23. $16\frac{1}{2}$	24. 9	25. 35
26. 78	27. 94	28. 99	29. $75\frac{1}{2}$	30. 89
31. $67\frac{1}{2}$	32. 44	33. 18	34. 14	35. $32\frac{1}{2}$
36. 47	37. 78	38. 190	39. 39	40. $85\frac{1}{2}$

PRACTICE SET A.1 ANSWERS

1. 440	2. 69	3. 2332	4. 774
5. 98	6. $22\frac{1}{2}$	7. 419	8. 959
9. 33	10. 44	11. 64	12. 98
13. 89	14. 16	15. 14	16. cccxlix
17. cmvi	18. li	19. mcdxcix	20. lxxxviiiss
21. lv	22. xxix	23. xviss	24. ix
25. xxxv	26. lxxviii	27. xciv	28. xcix
29. lxxvss	30. lxxxix	31. lxviiss	32. xliv
33. xviii	34. xiv	35. xxxiiss	36. xlvii
37. lxxviii	38. cxc	39. xxxix	40. lxxxvss

APPENDIX II
Commonly Used Medical Abbreviations*

Latin abbreviation	Latin words	Meaning
ā	ante	before
ac	ante cibum	before meals
ad lib	ad libitum	freely as desired
alt h	alternis horis	every other hour
aq	aqua	water
bid*	bis in die	twice a day
c̄	cum	with
cap	capsula	capsules
dil	dilue	dilute
h	hora	hour
hs	hora somni	bedtime
p	post	after
pc	post cibum	after meals
per	per	by
po or (PO)	per ora	by mouth
prn	pro re nata	when necessary
q	quaque	every, each
qd	quaque die	daily
qh	quaque hora	every hour
qid	quater in die	four times a day
qod	quaque otra die	every other day
q2h	quaque 2 horis	every 2 hours
r	rectalium	rectal
s̄s̄	semi	one-half
stat	statim	immediately
tab	tabula	tablet
tid	ter in die	three times a day

*Sometimes these abbreviations are written with periods; for example, b.i.d., q.i.d.

EXAMPLE A.6

Rewrite the following prescriptions using medical abbrevations.

(a) Camalox: 4 drams, four times a day, after meals and at bedtime.

Answer. Camalox: ʒ iv
qid pc & hs

(b) Propoxyphene HCL: 35 milligrams. Take two tablets every 6 hours as needed for pain.

Answer. Propoxyphene HCL: 35 mg
tab ii q6h prn

(c) PenVee K 300 milligrams per teaspoon: Give 1 teaspoon four times a day.

Answer. PenVee K 300 mg/tsp
1 tsp qid

EXAMPLE A.7

Rewrite the following directions using the meanings of the abbreviations.

(a) Maalox: Give fʒ ii alt hr

Answer. Maalox: Give 2 fluid drams every other hour.

(b) KCL: 10% soln, 15 mL bid

Answer. KCL: Give a 10% solution, 15 milliliters twice a day.

(c) Morphine sulfate gr $\frac{1}{4}$ IM q4h prn

Answer. Morphine sulfate: Administer $\frac{1}{4}$ grain intramuscularly every four hours as needed for pain.

PRACTICE SET A.2

Fill in the blanks.

1. _____ = $\bar{a}$
2. bid = _____
3. dil = _____
4. _____ = after meals
5. hs = _____

Rewrite the following directions using abbreviations.

6. Seconal Sodium: 25 milligrams, given intramuscularly at bedtime
7. Librium: 5 milligram capsules twice a day as needed for nerves
8. Codeine: 1 grain every 6 hours as needed for pain
9. Duracillin: 450 000 U IM A.M.
10. Chloromycetin: 50 milligrams IV q6h

Rewrite the following prescriptions using the meanings of the abbreviations.

11. Dyazide: cap ii bid
12. Serpasil: 500 mcg po qd
13. V-Cillin K: 400 000 U q6h
14. Gantrisin: 4 g po stat, then 2 g q4h
15. K-Lyte tabs: Dissolve tab i in f℥ vi aq stat

Rewrite the following prescriptions using the correct abbreviations.

16. Riboflavin: 10 milligrams by mouth, three times a day after meals
17. Elixir Terpin hydrate: 1 dram every four hours, as needed
18. Phenobarbital: 5 grains given intramuscularly every three hours
19. Prednisone: 7.5 mg by mouth four times a day
20. Keflex: 250 mg by mouth twice a day
21. Morphine: 10 milligrams given subcutaneously immediately
22. Thorazine: 15 milligrams given intramuscularly every six hours, as needed for pain
23. Seconal Sodium: 75 milligrams given intramuscularly at bedtime, as needed
24. Penicillin: 1.2 million units given intramuscularly every four hours
25. Lanoxin: 50 mcg by mouth daily

PRACTICE SET A.2 ANSWERS

1. before
2. twice a day
3. dilute
4. pc
5. bedtime
6. Seconal Sodium: 25 mg IM hs
7. Librium: 5 mg cap bid prn

Practice Set A.2 Answers

8. Codeine: gr i q6h prn
9. Duracillin: 450 000 units given intramuscularly before noon
10. Chloromycetin: 50 milligrams given intravenously every six hours
11. Dyazide capsules: 2 capsules twice a day
12. Serpasil: 500 micrograms by mouth daily
13. V-Cillin K: 400 000 units every six hours
14. Gantrisin: 4 grams by mouth immediately, then 2 grams every four hours
15. K-Lyte tablets: dissolve 1 tablet in 6 ounces of water and take immediately
16. Riboflavin: 10 mg po tid pc
17. Terpin Hydrate: ℨ i q4h prn
18. Phenobarbital: gr v IM q3h
19. Prednisone: 7.5 mg po qid
20. Keflex: 250 mg po bid
21. Morphine: 10 mg SC stat
22. Thorazine: 15 mg IM q6h prn
23. Seconal Sodium: 75 mg IM hs prn
24. Penicillin: 1.2 million U IM q4h
25. Lanoxin: 50 mcg po qd

APPENDIX III
West Nomogram

Appendix III. West Nomogram

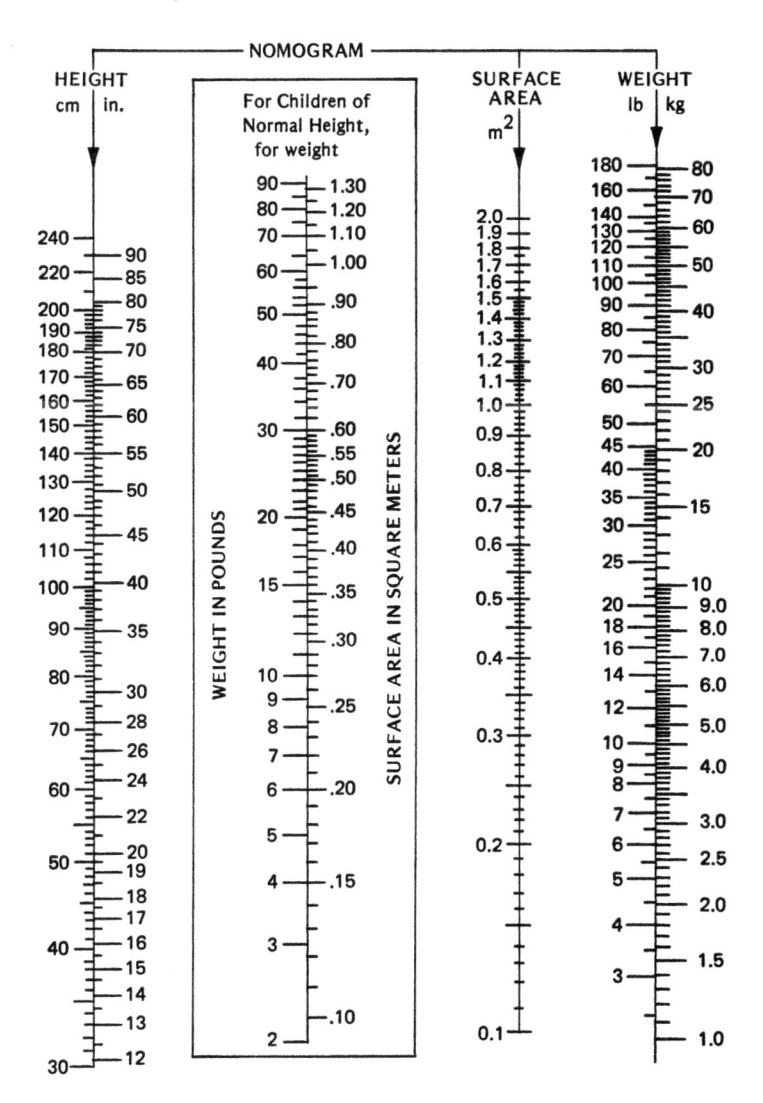

Figure A–1. West Nomogram. Draw a straight line connecting the height and weight of the patient. The number where the line intersects the surface area column is the patient's surface area. If a patient is of average size, use the column entitled "For Children of Normal Height, for weight." (Figure of West Nomogram modified from data of E. Boyd by C. D. West; from Victor C. Vaughn III, M.D. and R. James McKay, M.D., eds., *Nelson Textbook of Pediatrics*, 10th ed. [Philadelphia: W. B. Saunders Company, 1975], p. 1713. This and all other West Nomograms reprinted by permission of the publisher.)

APPENDIX IV
Final Exam Self Review

The Chapter 10 problems may be omitted if Chapter 10 is not part of the course.

Convert each of the following units as indicated.

Ch 5   1. f℥ xxxii = f℈ _____

Ch 4   2. 45 mL = _____ L

Ch 5   3. 5 glasses _____ oz

Ch 4   4. 0.70 g = _____ mcg

Ch 5   5. 14 in. = _____ cm

Ch 5   6. 11 tsp = _____ gtt

Ch 5   7. 105 mL = _____ oz

Ch 4   8. 0.08 kL = _____ L

Ch 4   9. 15 L = _____ cc

Ch 5   10. 3500 cc = _____ qt

Complete each of the following. Be sure to label each answer.

Ch 10   11. What is the percentage strength of a solution in which 90 g of a drug are dissolved in 1.5 liters of solution?

                                                               11. _____

Appendix IV.   Final Exam Self Review

Ch 10 **12.** How many mL of sterile solvent *should be added* to 350 mL of glycerin to make a 20% (V/V) solution?

12. _____

Ch 10 **13.** How many mL of 80% stock solution of isopropyl alcohol would you use to prepare 4 L of 50% isopropyl alcohol?

13. _____

Ch 7   **14.** A physician ordered 300 cc IV of a medicated solution. The patient is to receive 0.5 mL/min via a 60 gtt/mL administration set. Calculate the rate of flow.

14. _____

Ch 8   **15.** If the adult dose of sodium luminol is 100 mg, what is the dose for a 42-lb child?

15. _____

Ch 10 **16.** Prepare a 1:500 isopropyl alcohol solution from 1 L of 1% isopropyl alcohol. Preparation: _____

_____

Ch 7   **17.** Drug Order: IV mixture 3 g/L at a rate of 20 mcg/kg/min via a 60 gtt/mL administration set. Calculate the rate of flow for a 154-lb patient.

17. _____

Ch 6   **18.** Drug Order: 450 000 U Duracillin IM (Fig. A–2). Indicate by shading the syringe (Fig. A–3) how many mL you should administer.

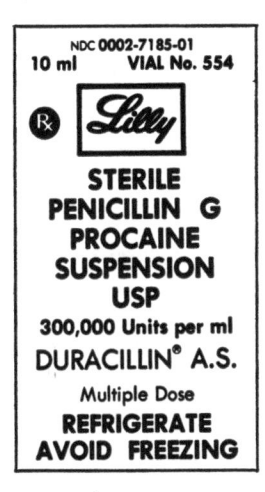

```
NDC 0002-7185-01
10 ml        VIAL No. 554

Rx   Lilly

STERILE
PENICILLIN G
PROCAINE
SUSPENSION
USP
300,000 Units per ml
DURACILLIN® A.S.
Multiple Dose
REFRIGERATE
AVOID FREEZING
```

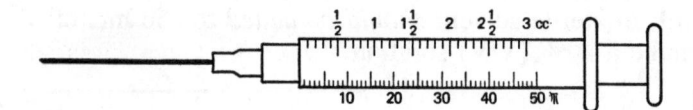

Figure A-3. 3 cc syringe

Ch 6 **19.** Drug Order: Phenobarbital gr $\frac{1}{2}$ tid. How many tabs will you give per dose (Fig. A–4)?

19. _____

Figure A-4. Phenobarbital

Ch 6 **20.** Write the administration for a patient who has been prescribed 500 mg of sodium ampicillin from a vial labeled, "1 g inject 2.4 mL of sterile water to yield 2.5 mL of sodium ampicillin solution." Administration: _____

_____

Ch 6 **21.** Administer 95 units of U-100 regular insulin using the 1 cc syringe (Fig. A–5). Indicate how much you would administer by shading in the correct amount.

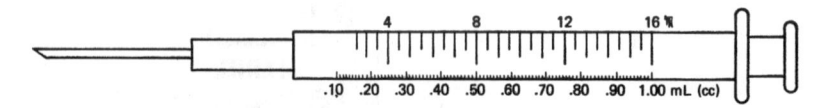

Figure A-5. 1 mL syringe

Ch 4 **22.** Convert 250°C to Fahrenheit temperature.

22. _____

Ch 10 **23.** Epinephrine 1:20 000 (W/V) solution is available for injection. The doctor prescribes 200 mcg to be administered for asthma. How many mL will you administer to a 275-lb patient?

23. _____

Appendix IV. Final Exam Self Review   243

Ch 10 **24.** Mannitol solution 75% (W/V) is available. An order asks for 1.5 g/kg body mass. How many mL will you administer to a 275-lb patient?

24. _____

Ch 8 **25.** Order: Bleomycin 2.5 U/m² body surface; available, reconstituted bleomycin 3.75 U/mL. How many mL will you administer to a patient with 1.88 m² body surface?

25. _____

Ch 8 **26.** Calculate the Garamycin dosage for a child with 0.86 m² body surface if the adult dose is 60 mg.

26. _____

Ch 8 **27.** Calculate the dosage of sulfisoxazole for a child who is 50 inches tall and who weighs 65 lb. The order is for 1.5 g/m² body surface.

27. _____

Ch 4 **28.** Convert 80°F to °C.

28. _____

Ch 10 **29.** A 0.0025% Merthiolate solution is needed for a wet dressing. How many mL of 0.0025% Merthiolate solution can be made from 0.25 mL of 1% solution?

29. _____

Ch 10 **30.** Order: gr $\frac{1}{250}$ of 0.05% (W/V) solution. How many ℳ should be administered?

30. _____

Ch 7 **31.** 1.5 L of packed cells are to be administered intravenously over 720 minutes, using a delivery set with a drop factor of 20 gtt/mL. What is the rate of flow?

31. _____

Ch 6 **32.** Drug Order: 450 units of U-500 diphtheria antitoxin. Shade in the syringe to indicate the correct amount to be administered (Fig. A–6).

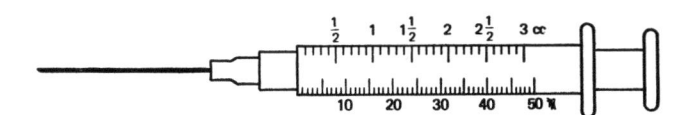

Figure A–6. 3 cc syringe

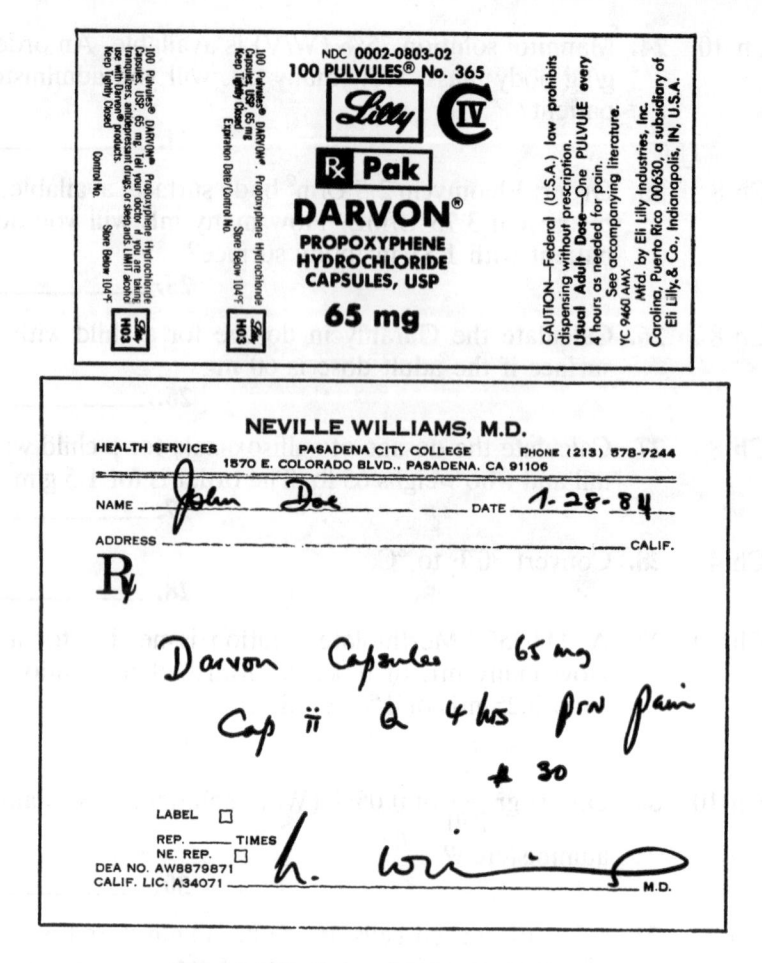

Figure A-7. Darvon and prescription

Ch 6   **33.** How many mg will be administered to the patient per dose (Fig. A-7)?

33. _____

Ch 5   **34.** Drug Order: Atropine gr $\frac{1}{400}$

Available: Atropine gr $\frac{1}{200}$ per ʒ

How many ʒ should be administered?

34. _____

Appendix IV.   Final Exam Self Review   245

Ch 5   **35.** A physician prescribed Klorvess 30 mEq dil in juice qd for a patient. On hand is Klorvess liquid solution 20 mEq/15 mL. How many mL should be administered?

35. _____

Ch 7   **36.** Ordered: 1000 mL of D5W IV over 8 hr. The administration set reads 25 gtt/mL. If after 4 hr only 400 mL have been delivered, calculate a new rate of flow so that the medication will be delivered in the eight hours.

36. _____

Ch 4   **37.** A patient is to receive 600 mcg digitoxin. The tablets on hand are 0.1 mg and 0.2 mg. Which strength and how many tablets should be administered?

37. _____

Ch 8   **38.** A doctor prescribes epinephrine for a patient who is 10 years old. The usual adult dose is 0.25 mg. How much should be administered?

38. _____

Ch 6   **39.** Order: Aramine 5000 mcg. How many mL should be administered (Fig. A–8)?

39. _____

Figure A–8. Aramine

Ch 10   **40.** Drug Order: 50 mg Methocarbamol IM. On hand is 1:15 (W/V) Methocarbamol solution. How many mL should be administered?

40. _____

Ch 9   **41.** Convert 3:00 P.M. to twenty-four hour clock time.

41. _____

Ch 9   **42.** Convert 2100 to traditional clock time.

42. _____

MEDICATION RECORD		NOTE:				
ADMINISTRATION PERIOD 07:01 03/13/87 to 07:00 03/14/87					A.M. SHIFT	P.M. SHIFT
NO	MEDICATION DOSE, FREQUENCY			START DATE / STOP DATE	0701 to 1500	1501 to 2300
SCH 19	URECHOLINE (BETHANECHOL) 10 MG TAB– 1 TAB + TID PO TOTAL DOSE = 15 MG			03/12/87 RENEW	09:00 13:00	17:00

Figure A–9. Medication administration record

Use Figure A–9 to answer questions 43 through 45.

Ch 9   **43.** At what times (traditional clock time) should the medication be administered?

43. _____

Ch 9   **44.** How many mg of Urecholine should be administered per dose? How many tablets is this?

44. _____

Ch 9   **45.** By what route and how often is this medication to be administered?

45. _____

APPENDIX V
Answers

DIAGNOSTIC TEST SOLUTION KEY

1. $38\frac{7}{10}$
2. $\frac{15}{16}$
3. $14\frac{23}{36}$
4. $7\frac{7}{8}$
5. $1\frac{1}{3}$
6. 0.3
7. 1.3
8. 0.8
9. 0.2
10. 2.4
11. 9.181
12. 8.2877
13. 2.16432
14. 3.255
15. 4500
16. 0.33%
17. 90%
18. 4%
19. 650%
20. 42.5%
21. 0.000025
22. 0.058
23. 0.035
24. 0.009
25. 3.15
26. $\frac{1}{3}$ or 0.33
27. $\frac{2}{25}$ or 0.08
28. 900
29. 80
30. $\frac{7}{400}$ or 0.0175
31. 0.005
32. $0.00\overline{6}$ or 0.007
33. $0.\overline{1}$ or 0.11
34. 0.0002
35. 0.125
36. 5.34

37. 3.87   **38.** 133.33 or $133\frac{1}{3}$ **39.** 18.75   **40.** 37.5%

41. 0.1%   **42.** 0.025%   **43.** 5%   **44.** 1:400

45. 2:300   **46.** $83\frac{1}{3}$ **47.** 25   **48.** 300

49. 102   **50.** 2

CHAPTER 1.

PRETEST

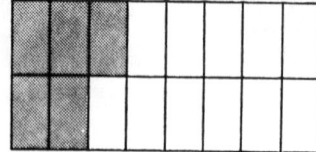

1.

2. $3\frac{3}{7}$ **3.** $\frac{75}{11}$ **4.** $\frac{6}{7}$ **5.** $\frac{25}{65}$

6. $\frac{11}{3}$ **7.** LCD = 420   **8.** $\frac{19}{24}$ **9.** $\frac{1}{2}$

10. $4\frac{3}{10}$ **11.** $2\frac{17}{24}$ **12.** 30   **13.** $\frac{2}{25}$

14. $\frac{1}{3}$ **15.** $\frac{8}{9}$

PRACTICE SET 1.1

1. (a) $\frac{6}{8}$ (b) $\frac{2}{6}$ **2.** $\frac{7}{12}$

   (c) $\frac{3}{16}$ (d) $\frac{4}{7}$

3. Numerator is 4; denominator is 9.

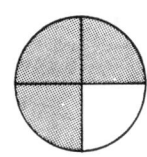

Appendix V. Practice Set 1.3   **249**

4. (a) [circle with 3/4 shaded]   (b) [rectangle 2×3 with 5/6 shaded]

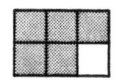

(c) [pentagon with 2/5 shaded]   (d) [bar with 10 segments, 6/10 shaded]

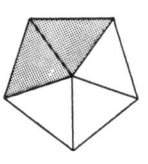

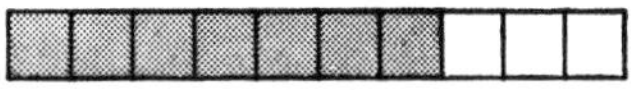

5. $\dfrac{4}{10}$ or $\dfrac{2}{5}$

PRACTICE SET 1.2

1. $\dfrac{16}{3}, \dfrac{5}{5}, \dfrac{11}{4}$ **2.** $4\dfrac{1}{2}, 5\dfrac{1}{3}, 2\dfrac{10}{11}, 1\dfrac{1}{7}, 3\dfrac{1}{5}$

3. $\dfrac{9}{4}, \dfrac{15}{8}, \dfrac{11}{2}, \dfrac{25}{4}, \dfrac{35}{4}$

4. (a) $\dfrac{5}{10}$ **5.** (a) $\dfrac{2}{3}$

(b) $\dfrac{27}{72}$ (b) $\dfrac{3}{8}$

(c) $\dfrac{100}{125}$ (c) $\dfrac{2}{3}$

PRACTICE SET 1.3

1. $\dfrac{12}{8} = 1\dfrac{1}{2}$ **2.** $\dfrac{10}{10} = 1$

3. $3\dfrac{7}{5} = 4\dfrac{2}{5}$ **4.** $3\dfrac{22}{16} = 4\dfrac{3}{8}$

5. $3\dfrac{10}{8} = 4\dfrac{1}{4}$ **6.** $\dfrac{4}{12} = \dfrac{1}{3}$

7. $\dfrac{9}{18} = \dfrac{1}{2}$

8. $2\dfrac{2}{10} = 2\dfrac{1}{5}$

9. $2\dfrac{2}{8} = 2\dfrac{1}{4}$

10. $2\dfrac{1}{15}$

11. LCD = 72; $\dfrac{3}{8}$

12. LCD = 120; $\dfrac{41}{120}$

13. LCD = 80; $\dfrac{1}{80}$

14. LCD = 45; $\dfrac{13}{45}$

15. LCD = 90; $\dfrac{53}{90}$

16. LCD = 40; $10\dfrac{7}{40}$

17. LCD = 6; $79\dfrac{1}{6}$

18. LCD = 40; $5\dfrac{1}{8}$

19. LCD = 60; $1\dfrac{19}{20}$

20. LCD = 60; $8\dfrac{7}{15}$

21. $\dfrac{1}{9}$

22. $\dfrac{4}{21}$

23. $\dfrac{1}{5}$

24. $\dfrac{10}{3} = 3\dfrac{1}{3}$

25. $\dfrac{15}{2} = 7\dfrac{1}{2}$

26. $\dfrac{2}{3}$

27. $\dfrac{3}{8}$

28. 36

29. 2

30. $\dfrac{25}{12} = 2\dfrac{1}{12}$

1.4 CHAPTER 1 REVIEW PROBLEMS

1. $\dfrac{5}{8}$

2. $\dfrac{6}{20}$ or $\dfrac{3}{10}$

3. $\dfrac{2}{5}$

4. $\dfrac{12}{20}$ or $\dfrac{3}{5}$

5. $\dfrac{6}{10}$ or $\dfrac{3}{5}$

6. Denominator = 5

Appendix V. 1.4 Chapter 1 Review Problems

7. $4\frac{1}{2}$

8. $2\frac{6}{11}$

9. $5\frac{2}{3}$

10. $4\frac{1}{5}$

11. 4

12. $1\frac{4}{5}$

13. $12\frac{1}{10}$

14. $11\frac{3}{8}$

15. $12\frac{8}{11}$

16. $6\frac{11}{20}$

17. $\frac{7}{4}$

18. $\frac{13}{9}$

19. $\frac{27}{5}$

20. $\frac{25}{4}$

21. $\frac{11}{3}$

22. $\frac{23}{8}$

23. $\frac{42}{10}$

24. $\frac{20}{3}$

25. $\frac{35}{4}$

26. $\frac{49}{5}$

27. $\frac{10}{20}$

28. $\frac{20}{24}$

29. $\frac{63}{72}$

30. $\frac{40}{100}$

31. $\frac{21}{24}$

32. $\frac{2}{3}$

33. $\frac{3}{4}$

34. $\frac{5}{6}$

35. Cannot be reduced

36. $\frac{2}{5}$

37. $\frac{7}{8}$

38. $\frac{17}{19}$

39. $\frac{4}{7}$

40. $\frac{1}{3}$

41. $\frac{13}{15}$

42. $\frac{8}{10} = \frac{4}{5}$

43. $\frac{2}{8} = \frac{1}{4}$

44. LCD = 24; $\frac{19}{24}$

45. LCD = 72; $\frac{13}{72}$

46. LCD = 24; $\frac{5}{8}$

47. LCD = 48; $\frac{49}{48} = 1\frac{1}{48}$

48. LCD = 8; $3\frac{5}{8}$

49. LCD = 15; $12\frac{14}{15}$

50. LCD = 56; $1\frac{53}{56}$

51. LCD = 32; $3\frac{23}{32}$

52. $\frac{2}{5}$ 53. $\frac{1}{3}$ 54. $8\frac{1}{4}$

55. $15\frac{1}{2}$ 56. 57 57. $1\frac{1}{2}$

58. 9 59. 6 60. $2\frac{2}{3}$

CHAPTER 2

PRETEST

1. Four thousand three and sixty-five ten thousandths
2. 340.00340
3. Hundredths place
4. 31.098
5. 1.90
6. 28.136
7. 27.317
8. 0.00045
9. 4.1
10. 35
11. 708
12. 0.3
13. 1.125
14. 2.748 kg
15. 7.11 kg

PRACTICE SET 2.1

1. Hundredths place; five and fifteen thousandths
2. Ones place; thirteen and five tenths
3. Hundreds place; one thousand, four hundred ninety-seven and nine hundred ten thousandths
4. Ten thousandths; one hundred seven hundred thousandths
5. Hundred thousands place; nine million, five hundred six thousand and nine hundredths
6. 62.0525
7. 13.02
8. 0.00137
9. 2,025.000006
10. 9,050,002.006

PRACTICE SET 2.2

1. 1.2
2. 0.99
3. 4.50
4. 1.440, 1.401, 1.4, 1.0440
5. 0.201, 0.2, 0.0222, 0.020
6. 2.8
7. 4.50
8. 0.0016
9. 8
10. 5654

PRACTICE SET 2.3

1. 174.172
2. 50.86
3. 184.571
4. 14.79
5. 48.152
6. 7.71
7. 0.02744
8. 0.975
9. 30.6324
10. 6.25
11. 3.32
12. 24.7
13. 34.1
14. 4766
15. 6.65

PRACTICE SET 2.4

1. 0.875
2. 0.6
3. 9.75
4. 0.56
5. 1.429
6. $\frac{3}{20}$
7. $\frac{3}{8}$
8. $\frac{1}{8}$
9. $\frac{4}{5}$
10. $\frac{1}{16}$

2.5 CHAPTER 2 REVIEW PROBLEMS

1. Thousandths place
2. Tenths place
3. Thousands place
4. Hundred thousandths place
5. Millions place
6. Nine thousand, six hundred seven and five hundredths

7. Thirteen and sixty-five ten thousandths
8. Ninety-one hundred thousandths
9. Three and five hundred millionths
10. One million, four thousand, seven and nine tenths
11. 0.037
12. 3.000115
13. 2 041.06
14. 1 200 000.5
15. 27 003.0004
16. 3.333, 3.33, 3.0330, 3.0033
17. 1.100, 1.011, 1.01, 1.001
18. 10.999, 10.99, 10.9, 10.099

19. 16.1	20. 90	21. 356.56
22. 414	23. 0.051	24. 516,914.092
25. 1.0014	26. 45.411	27. 520.117
28. 97.701	29. 9.23	30. 496.84
31. 0.307	32. 0.0287	33. 96
34. 0.00009648	35. 44.30	36. 9.13
37. 2234.8	38. 0.125	39. 1.17
40. 2.083	41. 21 days	42. 150 grams
43. 1.575 grams	44. 33.6 milligrams	45. 2.675 milligrams
46. $\frac{1}{4}$	47. 3.86	

CHAPTER 3.

PRETEST

1. $0.3:100; \dfrac{0.3}{100}$
2. $46\dfrac{2}{3}$

Appendix V. Practice Set 3.3   255

3. 50

5. 30%

7. 250

9. 13.8 milligrams

4. 0.0385

6. $6\frac{2}{25}$

8. 8 liters

10. 175 persons

PRACTICE SET 3.1

1. 10:12; $\frac{10}{12}$

2. $3\frac{1}{2}:1$; $\frac{3\frac{1}{2}}{1}$

3. 10 mg:1 lb; $\frac{10 \text{ mg}}{1 \text{ lb}}$

4. 8 oz:1 glass; $\frac{8 \text{ oz}}{1 \text{ glass}}$

5. 45 mL:12 hr; $\frac{45 \text{ mL}}{12 \text{ hr}}$

6. 455 = 455; True

7. 35 = 35; True

8. 45 ≠ 54; False

9. 34.4 = 34.4; True

10. 6.28 = 6.28; True

PRACTICE SET 3.2

1. $x = 65$

2. $x = 39$

3. $x = 33\frac{1}{3}$

4. $x = 66\frac{2}{3}$

5. $x = 6$

6. $\frac{4}{5}$ or 0.8 mL

7. $\frac{1}{3}$ or 0.33 mL

PRACTICE SET 3.3

1. 0.37

2. 0.82

3. 4

4. 0.005

5. $0.12\frac{3}{4}$ or 0.1275

6. $0.62\frac{1}{2}$ or 0.625

7. 0.008
8. 0.386
9. 0.0027
10. 0.0008
11. 0.0005
12. 0.00025
13. 0.75

PRACTICE SET 3.4

1. % = x%   W = 500   P = 10
2. % = 35%   W = x   P = 42
3. % = 0.6%   W = 44   P = x
4. x = 1166.7
5. x = 20%
6. $\frac{1}{2}$ kg
7. $\frac{1}{2}$ mL
8. $\frac{1}{2}$ oz
9. $\frac{1}{2}$ liter
10. 5 people

3.5 CHAPTER 3 REVIEW PROBLEMS

1. 8:5; $\frac{8}{5}$
2. 7.3:1; $\frac{7.3}{1}$
3. $2\frac{1}{2}$:100; $\frac{2\frac{1}{2}}{100}$
4. 100 mg:1 mL; $\frac{100 \text{ mg}}{1 \text{ mL}}$
5. 6 g:1 m²; $\frac{6g}{1 \text{ m}^2}$
6. True
7. True
8. False
9. 65
10. 70
11. 0.9 or $\frac{15}{16}$
12. 1.5
13. 37
14. 105
15. 0.3 or $\frac{1}{3}$
16. 1.5 oz
17. 1.3 or $1\frac{1}{4}$ cc
18. 0.7 mL
19. 21.8 or $21\frac{3}{4}$ g
20. 7.7 mg
21. 0.14

Appendix V.   Practice Set 4.3

22. 0.06
23. 0.007
24. 0.0002
25. 0.158
26. 47%
27. 3%
28. 350%
29. 728%
30. 0.82%
31. 130
32. 33.3 or $33\frac{1}{3}$%
33. 63
34. 20%
35. 56
36. 15 people
37. 165 people
38. 75 parts
39. 0.1 part
40. 0.25 part

CHAPTER 4.

PRACTICE SET 4.1

1. 1 kg
2. 1 mcL
3. 1 cm
4. 1 mm
5. 1 dag
6. 0.1 g
7. 0.000001 L
8. 0.001 m
9. 1000 m
10. 10 g
11. 100 cg
12. 1000 mL

PRACTICE SET 4.2

1. 50 000 mg
2. 0.003 m
3. 2 L
4. 0.0012 kg
5. 140 000 000 mcm
6. 600 mcg
7. 3460 dag
8. 0.1416 m
9. 0.001678 m
10. 50 g

PRACTICE SET 4.3

1. 140°F
2. 250°C
3. 10°C
4. 110.3°F
5. 52°C

PRACTICE SET 4.4

1. tab erythromycin (0.25g/tab)
2. 1.3 cc
3. 2.7 g Flagyl
4. 10.5 cc indocyanine green
5. Use one 600 mg tab and one 300 mg tab sodium bicarbonate (or three 300 mg tabs).

4.5 CHAPTER 4 REVIEW PROBLEMS

1. 150°C
2. 3250 mL
3. 1 mcL
4. 8.5432 daL
5. 7.95 g
6. 0.035 g
7. 5500 cm^3
8. 140°F
9. 250 mL
10. 0.0019 L
11. 54.4°C
12. 4.5 g
13. 5 000 000 mm
14. 163.76°F
15. 0.395 L
16. 59 000 cc
17. 0.0000145 L
18. 30°C
19. 482°F
20. 2 mL
21. 0.0016 kL
22. 0.8 cm
23. 9.54 kg
24. 1000 mL
25. 1 L
26. 2 tabs Deltasone (10 mg/tab)
27. 15 cc Gantrisin syrup
28. 2 tabs magnesium carbonate (0.2 g/tab)
29. $5\frac{1}{3}$ cc hydrocodone bitartrate
30. 2 tabs sodium bicarbonate (600 mg/tab)
31. 2 tabs aspirin (450 mg/tab)
32. 2 cc
33. 1.5 tabs
34. 3 tabs methionine
35. Use one 4 mg tab and one 3.5 mg tab methyclothiazide
36. 5 tabs
37. 1 tab methionine (200 mg/tab)
38. 1 tab methyclothiazide (3.5 mg/tab)

Appendix V. Practice Set 5.3

39. 18 cc Gantrisin syrup

40. 2 tabs diphemanil methylsulfate (250 mg/tab)

CHAPTER 5.

PRACTICE SET 5.1

1. ℳ cdl	**2.** qt ix	**3.** gr mxxiv	**4.** f℥ ccxl
5. ℨ dcclxiv	**6.** gal xxviii	**7.** f℥ cmvi	**8.** ℨ lxxxviiiss
9. ℨ xliii	**10.** ℳ lxxv	**11.** pt vi	**12.** gr $\frac{1}{50}$
13. f℥ iiss	**14.** lb lix	**15.** ℳ cxvi	**16.** f℥ xcv
17. ℨ xvii	**18.** gr $\frac{1}{250}$	**19.** gal iv	**20.** qt xxxix

PRACTICE SET 5.2

1. 10 oz	**2.** 150 gtt	**3.** 5 tbsp	**4.** 15 tsp	**5.** 35 oz
6. 41 gtt	**7.** 9 tsp	**8.** 12 tbsp	**9.** 10 gtt	**10.** 11 oz

PRACTICE SET 5.3

1. ℨ ivss	**2.** ℳ mmmdcccxl	**3.** qt i	**4.** f℥ iiss
5. ℨ iii	**6.** ℳ mcmxx	**7.** pt iv	**8.** f℥ ccclxxxiv
9. f℥ v	**10.** f℥ i	**11.** 2 tsp	**12.** $5\frac{1}{2}$ glasses
13. $\frac{1}{2}$ oz	**14.** 900 gtt	**15.** 80 tbsp	**16.** 16 tbsp
17. $13\frac{1}{2}$ tsp	**18.** $4\frac{3}{4}$ glasses	**19.** 18 tsp	**20.** $112\frac{1}{2}$ gtt

PRACTICE SET 5.4

1. 5.4 in.
2. ℥ cxiiss
3. 45 mg
4. 33 lb
5. 60 mL
6. $\frac{1}{2}$ g
7. $5\frac{1}{2}$ tsp
8. $\frac{1}{2}$ tbsp
9. $\frac{3}{4}$ cc
10. ℥ vi
11. 24 oz
12. 2 tbsp
13. $\frac{1}{2}$ tab
14. 6 doses
15. ʒ iv
16. 1 tab (600 mg/tab)
17. $1\frac{1}{2}$ mL
18. 2 tbsp
19. $3\frac{1}{2}$ mL
20. 2.1 grams/dose

5.5 CHAPTER 5 REVIEW PROBLEMS

1. 424 ounces
2. $69\frac{1}{2}$ pints
3. $27\frac{1}{2}$ grains
4. 1560 pounds
5. 72 gallons
6. fʒ cdxii
7. ℥ dccxxv
8. pt lxxxss
9. qt xlii
10. gr mcxl
11. ʒ ccxxi
12. gr xc
13. ʒ iiss
14. ʒ iv
15. ʒ xxiv
16. 450 gtt
17. 40 tbsp
18. $\frac{3}{4}$ glass
19. 2 tbsp
20. 9 tbsp
21. ℥ ccxl
22. ʒ xxxvi
23. ʒ ss
24. ℥ dc
25. 7500 mL
26. 15 g
27. $39\frac{3}{5}$ lb
28. fʒ ivss
29. ℥ lx
30. 48 tbsp
31. $5\frac{1}{2}$ glasses
32. $5\frac{1}{2}$ liters
33. 59.1 in.
34. ℥ xxiv
35. ʒ v
36. ℥ xiv
37. 2 capsules
38. 32 doses
39. 3 tabs (gr iss tabs)

Appendix V. Practice Set 6.2

40. 8 tabs
41. 2 tabs
42. ℳ x
43. 12 doses
44. 5 glasses
45. 3 tbsp
46. $2\frac{2}{3}$ days
47. 18 tsp
48. 1.9 mL
49. $\frac{1}{2}$ tsp (approximately)
50. $2\frac{1}{2}$ oz

CHAPTER 6.

PRACTICE SET 6.1

1. 5 caps Colace (50 mg/tab)
2. 600 mg potassium chloride
3. 2 tabs pancreatin (325 mg/tab)
4. 4 tabs Tegopen (250 mg/tab)
5. 2 tabs Achromycin (250 mg/cap)
6. 2 tabs phenobarbital (gr $\frac{1}{4}$/tab)
7. 2 tabs Tylenol (300 mg/tab)
8. 2 tabs codeine (gr $\frac{1}{3}$/tab)
9. 3 tabs penicillin G potassium per dose (500 000 U/tab)
10. 5 tabs penicillin G potassium (100 000 U/tab) per dose

PRACTICE SET 6.2

1. 3 mL drug (0.05 mg/mL)
2. 12 mL Vibramycin (25 mg/ʒ)
3. 150 mg Keflex
4. 10 mL Ilosone (125 mg/5 mL)

5. 1 cc Betalin 12 Crystalline (100 mcg/mL)
6. ℨ vi KCl (20 mEq/ℨ)
7. 8 mg Lasix
8. 10 mL chloral hydrate (250 mg/5 mL)
9. 6.4 mL sulfadiazine (250 mg/L)
10. 10 mL hydrocodone bitartrate (2 mg/5 mL)

PRACTICE SET 6.3

1. Inject 1.8 mL of sterile water into the Staphcillin vial and shake well to dissolve; withdraw 1.6 mL and administer.
2. 0.5 mL heparin (40 000 U/mL)
3. 0.7 mL morphine sulfate (gr$\frac{1}{4}$/mL) (Fig. A–10)

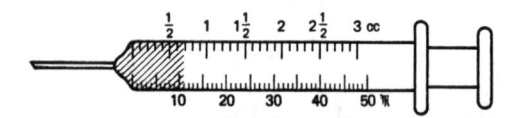

Figure A–10. 3 cc syringe

4. 0.5 mL penicillin G potassium (250 000 U/mL)
5. 1 cc sodium luminal (130 mg/2 mL) (Fig. A–11)

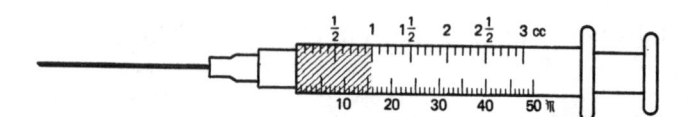

Figure A–11. 3 cc syringe

6. 0.6 mL Demerol (0.05 g/mL)
7. 3 mL penicillin G potassium
8. 0.6 mL U-100 isophane insulin (Fig. A–12)

Appendix V. 6.4 Chapter 6 Review Problems 263

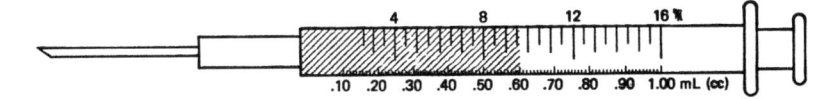

Figure A–12. 1 mL syringe

9. 70 units U-100 NPH Iletin (Fig. A–13)

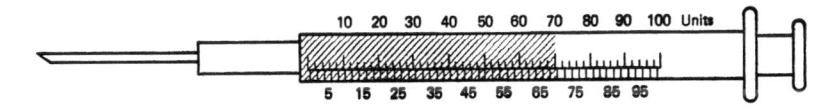

Figure A–13. 100 U syringe

10. 0.5 mL U-500 insulin (Fig. A–14)

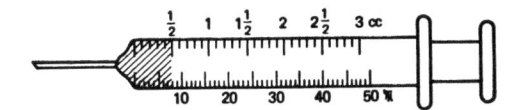

Figure A–14. 3 cc syringe

6.4 CHAPTER 6 REVIEW PROBLEMS

1. 0.45 mL U-100 insulin (Fig. A–15)

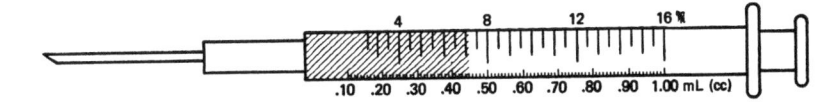

Figure A–15. 1 mL syringe

2. One Vitamin A tab (50 U/tab) per dose
3. 1.5 cc Crysticillin (300 000 U/cc)
4. 0.5 mL U-500 insulin (Fig. A–16)

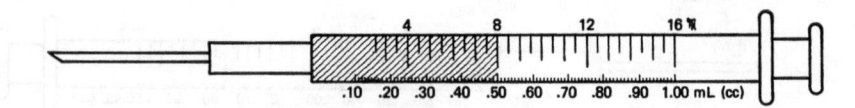

Figure A–16. 1 mL syringe

5. 22.5 mL Klorvess (20 mEq/15 mL)
6. 20 tabs V-Cillin K (250 mg tab)
7. 0.75 mL U-100 insulin (Fig. A–17)

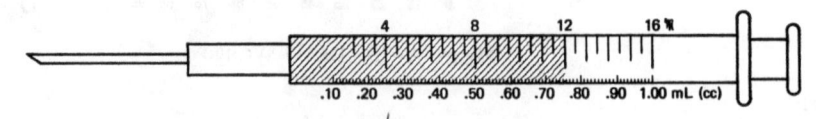

Figure A–17. 1 mL syringe

8. 1.5 mL penicillin G (Fig. A–18)

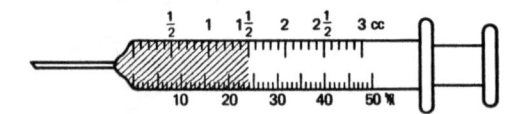

Figure A–18. 3 cc syringe

9. 2.7 mL bleomycin (10 U/mL)
10. 3 tabs Thyroid (gr $\overline{ss}$/tab)
11. 1.2 mL morphine (10 mg/mL)
12. 0.4 cc atropine sulfate (0.3 g/2 cc)
13. 5 mL sodium bicarbonate (gr v/5 mL)
14. Inject 2.4 mL of sterile water into 1 g vial of sodium ampicillin and shake well to dissolve; withdraw 1.25 mL and administer.
15. 0.6 mL regular insulin (Fig. A–19)

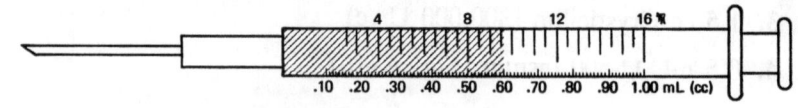

Figure A–19. 1 mL syringe

Appendix V. 6.4 Chapter 6 Review Problems

16. 0.78 mL penicillin G potassium (Fig. A–20)

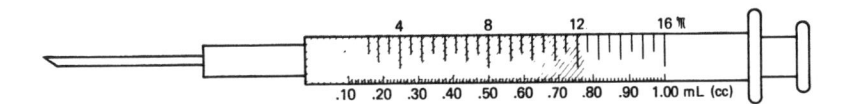

Figure A–20. 1 mL syringe

17. 1.8 mL bleomycin (10 U/mL)
18. 1.4 mL Drolban (50 mg/mL)
19. 3 caps Benadryl (50 mg/cap)
20. 2 capsules Darvon
21. 4 caps Nembutal (gr $\frac{3}{4}$/cap)
22. 3 tabs aspirin (300 mg/tab)
23. 2 tabs Stilbestrol (25 mg/tab)
24. 0.37 mL (Fig. A–21)

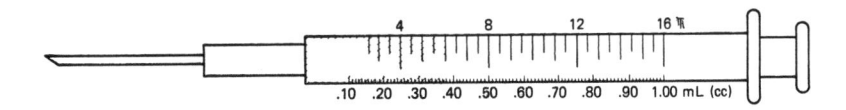

Figure A–21. 1 mL syringe

25. 0.9 mL meperidine hydrochloride (25 mg/0.5 mL) (Fig. A–22)

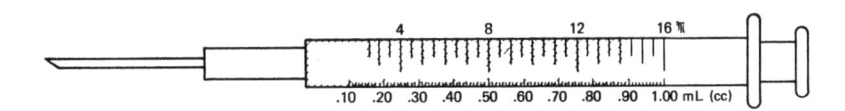

Figure A–22. 1 mL syringe

26. $2\frac{1}{2}$ mL penicillin G potassium (200 000 U/mL)

27. $1\frac{1}{4}$ mL heparin (40 000 U/mL)

28. 1 mL Demerol (100 mg/2 mL)

29. Inject 2.5 mL of sterile water in Loridine vial and shake well to dissolve; withdraw 2 mL and administer.

30. $1\frac{1}{4}$ mL atropine sulfate (0.4 mg/mL)

31. 1.5 cc Crysticillin (300 000 U/cc)

32. 0.4 mL digoxin (0.5 mg/2 mL)

33. 4 tablets Neotrizine stat; 2 tablets Neotrizine q6h

34. 2.4 mL heparin (Fig. A–23)

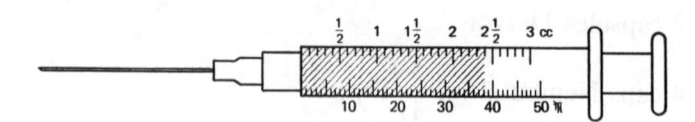

Figure A–23. 3 cc syringe

35. 0.75 mL U-500 insulin (Fig. A–24)

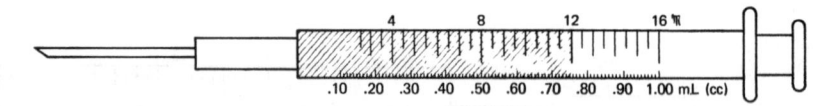

Figure A–24. 1 mL syringe

36. 0.55 mL U-100 insulin (Fig. A–25)

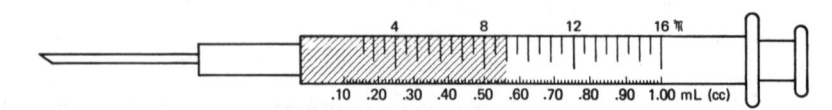

Figure A–25. 1 mL syringe

37. 0.4 mL ampicillin (125 mg/mL)

38. ℞ xx Dilaudid (3 mg/mL)

39. 15 mL KCl (40 mEq/30 mL)

CHAPTER 7.

PRACTICE SET 7.1

1. 25 gtt/min
2. 25 gtt/min
3. 50 gtt/min
4. 42 gtt/min
5. 42 gtt/min
6. 200 gtt/min
7. 30 gtt/min
8. 13 gtt/min
9. 67 gtt/min
10. 17 gtt/min
11. 12 gtt/min
12. 10 gtt/min
13. 21 gtt/min
14. 30 gtt/min
15. 11 gtt/min

PRACTICE SET 7.2

1. 600 min
2. 600 min
3. 364 min
4. 500 min
5. 800 min
6. 330 min
7. 660 min
8. 900 min
9. 120 min
10. 500 min

PRACTICE SET 7.3

1. 26 gtt/min
2. 52 gtt/min
3. 11 gtt/min
4. 22 gtt/min
5. 50 gtt/min
6. 131 min
7. 1425 min

7.4 CHAPTER 7 REVIEW PROBLEMS

1. 21 gtt/min
2. 100 gtt/min
3. 450 min
4. 17 gtt/min
5. 42 min
6. 26 gtt/min
7. 25 gtt/min
8. 63 gtt/min
9. 300 min
10. 10 gtt/min
11. 21 gtt/min
12. 480 min
13. 63 gtt/min
14. 37 gtt/min
15. 45 gtt/min
16. 150 gtt/min
17. 313 min
18. 133 gtt/min
19. 22 gtt/min; 66 mL
20. 58 gtt/min; 350 mL

CHAPTER 8.

PRACTICE SET 8.1

1. 13 mg Demerol
2. 3.8 gr aspirin
3. 15.6 mg tetracycline
4. 0.23 m²
5. 0.003 gr atropine
6. 3.9 mg Atarax
7. 2.7 g sulfisoxazole
8. 264 mcg epinephrine
9. 0.78 m²
10. 168 mg chloral hydrate

PRACTICE SET 8.2

1. 90 000 U penicillin
2. 13.6 mg phenobarbital
3. 5.5 mg Demerol
4. ℞ i Fowler's solution
5. 0.25 mL tincture of digitalis
6. 1.2 mg phenobarbital
7. 1 mg Vitamin K
8. 1.4 mL Milk of Magnesia
9. 176.8 mg Tempra
10. 240 mg

8.3 CHAPTER 8 REVIEW PROBLEMS

1. 6 mg phenobarbital
2. 86.7 mg Keflin
3. ℞ iv tincture of digitalis
4. 3 mg adrenalin
5. 0.2 mg morphine
6. 99.4 mg chloral hydrate
7. 0.001 gr atropine sulfate
8. 5.4 mg Nembutal
9. 250 mg sulfadiazine
10. 1.16 m²
11. 102.9 mg erythromycin
12. 1 cc castor oil
13. 1.9 mg epinephrine
14. 124 855.5 or 125 000 U penicillin
15. 16 mg hydrocodone bitartrate

CHAPTER 9.

PRACTICE SET 9.1

1. 0100
2. 1400
3. 1800
4. 1100
5. 1300
6. 2300
7. 0500
8. 2100
9. 2400
10. 2000
11. 0600
12. 1200
13. 1500
14. 0200
15. 2200
16. 9:00 P.M.
17. 2:00 A.M.
18. 7:00 A.M.
19. 1:00 P.M.
20. 1:00 A.M.
21. 4:00 P.M.
22. 8:00 P.M.
23. 3:00 P.M.
24. 5:00 A.M.
25. 6:00 P.M.
26. 8:00 A.M.
27. 12:00 A.M.
28. 7:00 P.M.
29. 5:00 P.M.
30. 2:00 P.M.

PRACTICE SET 9.2

1. Methyldopa
2. March 12, 1987
3. 9:00 A.M., 1:00 P.M., and 5:00 P.M.
4. 5
5. 250 mg
6. 5 mg tablets
7. No

8. Trazodone
9. 9:00 A.M. and 6:00 P.M.
10. 10:00 P.M.
11. 50 mg tablets
12. June 1, 1987
13. $1\frac{1}{2}$ tablets
14. No
15. 25 mg
16. Anacin-3
17. Every 4 hours as needed
18. IV
19. Every 6 hours
20. 325 mg tablets

9.3 CHAPTER 9 REVIEW PROBLEMS

1. 1400
2. 1900
3. 1200
4. 0900
5. 2300
6. 10:00 P.M.
7. 3:00 A.M.
8. 5:00 P.M.
9. 1:00 P.M.
10. 8:00 P.M.
11. Tocainide
12. 50 mg
13. Every 8 hours by injection as needed
14. Every 4 hours as needed for pain
15. 50 mg
16. Diphenhydramine
17. 400 mg
18. 8
19. Tonocard and Transderm-nitro
20. 5

Appendix V. Practice Set 10.1

CHAPTER 10.

PRACTICE SET 10.1

	Metric	*Apothecaries'*
1.	$\dfrac{1 \text{ g}}{20\,000 \text{ mL}}$	$\dfrac{1 \text{ gr}}{20\,000 \text{ ℳ}}$
2.	$\dfrac{60 \text{ mL}}{100 \text{ mL}}$ (can be any unit)	$\dfrac{60 \text{ drams}}{100 \text{ drams}}$
3.	$\dfrac{1 \text{ ml}}{1000 \text{ mL}}$ (can be any unit)	$\dfrac{1 \text{ ounce}}{1000 \text{ ounces}}$
4.	$\dfrac{0.3 \text{ g}}{100 \text{ mL}}$	$\dfrac{0.3 \text{ gr}}{100 \text{ ℳ}}$
5.	$\dfrac{10 \text{ g}}{100 \text{ mL}}$	$\dfrac{10 \text{ gr}}{100 \text{ ℳ}}$
6.	$\dfrac{1 \text{ g}}{20 \text{ mL}}$	$\dfrac{1 \text{ gr}}{20 \text{ ℳ}}$
7.	$\dfrac{1 \text{ mL}}{10 \text{ mL}}$ (can be any unit)	$\dfrac{1 \text{ ʒ}}{10 \text{ ʒ}}$
8.	$\dfrac{50 \text{ cc}}{100 \text{ cc}}$ (can be any unit)	$\dfrac{50 \text{ ℳ}}{100 \text{ ℳ}}$

9. 150 mg acetaminophen is dissolved in a 5 mL solution.

10. $\dfrac{0.6 \text{ g camphor}}{30 \text{ mL alcohol}}$

PRACTICE SET 10.2

1. 40 g boric acid crystals
2. 100 mL; take 2 g of sodium perborate and add enough sterile water to make exactly 100 mL.
3. 100 cc
4. Take 0.03 g of Ceepryn chloride and add enough sterile solvent to make exactly 150 mL.
5. 0.99 g; take 0.99 g of sodium chloride and add enough sterile solvent to make exactly 110 mL.
6. Take 2 mL of vinegar and add enough sterile solvent to make exactly 200 mL.
7. Take $13\frac{3}{4}$ g of magnesium sulfate and add enough sterile solvent to make exactly 250 mL.
8. 41.8 mg Feosol elixir
9. 2.5 mL Methocarbamol
10. Take 0.05 g of silver nitrate and add enough sterile solvent to make exactly 1 L.
11. 2.5 L Burow's solution.
12. 25 g of crystalline glucose; take 25 g of crystalline glucose and add enough sterile solvent to make exactly 500 mL.
13. 30 g of sodium bicarbonate; take 30 g of sodium bicarbonate and add enough sterile solvent to make exactly 300 mL.
14. 4 mL. Take 4 mL of silver nitrate and add enough sterile solvent to make exactly 200 mL.
15. 6250 drams of Burow's solution.
16. Add 150 mL of sterile solvent to the 50 mL of glycerin.
17. $18\frac{1}{3}$ mL Mercurochrome (15 mg/1 mL)
18. 2 750 mg sodium bicarbonate
19. 35 g dextrose and 3.5 g sodium chloride
20. 240 mL mannitol solution (25%)

Appendix V. Practice Set 10.4

PRACTICE SET 10.3

1. 1.5%
2. 0.5%; 1:200
3. 1.5%; 3:200
4. 4%; 1:25
5. 1.5%; 3:200; 1500 mg/100 mL sodium bromide solution
6. 5%
7. 1:50
8. 10%; 1:10
9. 1:5; $\dfrac{50 \text{ g Epsom salts}}{250 \text{ mL sterile water}}$
10. 2.5%; 1:40

PRACTICE SET 10.4

1. 10 mL of 1:10 potassium permanganate; take 10 mL of 1:10 potassium permanganate solution and add enough sterile solvent to make exactly 1000 mL.
2. 250 mL of 1:2 creosol solution; take 250 mL of 1:2 creosol solution and add enough sterile solvent to make exactly 500 mL.
3. 2500 mL of 1% formaldehyde solution
4. Add 0.3 gal of sterile water.
5. 150 mL of 6% sodium chloride solution
6. 0.4 mL of 25% solution; take 0.4 mL of the 25% solution and add enough sterile solvent to make exactly 500 mL.
7. 40 mL of 0.1% Ceepryn chloride; take 40 mL of 0.1% Ceepryn chloride and add enough sterile solvent to make exactly 200 mL.
8. $13\frac{1}{3}$ mL of 75% formaldehyde solution; take $13\frac{1}{3}$ mL of 75% formaldehyde solution and add enough sterile solvent to make exactly 1000 mL.
9. Add 200 mL of sterile solvent.
10. 1.5 mL of 5% cupric sulfate solution; take 1.5 mL of 5% cupric sulfate solution and add enough sterile solvent to make exactly 300 mL.
11. Take 225 mL of 0.2% nitrofurazone and add enough sterile solvent to make exactly 450 mL.

12. Take 40 mL of 1:1000 Zephiran Chloride and add enough sterile water to make exactly 800 mL.

13. 2 mL 5% cupric sulfate solution

14. 250 mL solvent

15. 20 mL of 1:20 sodium bicarbonate solution

10.5 CHAPTER 10 REVIEW PROBLEMS

1. Take 10 mL of 5% cupric sulfate solution and add enough sterile solvent to make exactly 200 mL.

2. 4 g of sodium perborate

3. 0.05%

4. Take 200 g of sodium chloride and add enough sterile solvent to make exactly 800 mL.

5. Take 100 mL of 6% acetic acid solution and add enough sterile solvent to make exactly 200 mL.

6. $33\frac{1}{3}$ mL of silver nitrate solution

7. 3 mL of gynergen tartrate

8. Add 23 mL of water to 460 mg of codeine sulfate.

9. 4%; 1:25

10. 30 g sodium chloride

11. Take 100 mL of $2\frac{1}{2}$% dextrose solution and add enough sterile solvent to make exactly 500 mL.

12. Take 30 mL of 0.1% Ceepryn chloride and add enough sterile solvent to make exactly 150 mL.

13. 5 g

14. 0.05%; 1:2000

15. 1000 mL of 50% alcohol

16. 12 g iodine crystals

17. 80 mL of 25% formaldehyde

Appendix V. 10.5 Chapter 10 Review Problems

18. ʒ cdl of glucose solution

19. 0.3%

20. Add $\frac{3}{4}$ L sterile water.

21. ℳ xxv of 0.04% solution

22. 10%

23. 250 mL of 3% Argyrol solution

24. 7.5 gtt potassium iodide (75%)

25. $3\frac{1}{3}$ mL of oxethazaine

26. Administer 125 gtt salicylate.

27. Take 8 tabs of mercuric chloride (gr viiss/tab) and add enough sterile solvent to make exactly 5 gal.

28. ℳ d of 1:1000 (W/V) solution

29. $3\frac{1}{3}$ mL of 75% magnesium sulfate

30. 102.3 mL of 1:500 epinephrine

31. 1.5%; 3:200

32. Take 125 g of sodium bicarbonate and add enough sterile solvent to make exactly 625 mL.

33. 1:200

34. Add fʒ ccxcviiiss of water to fʒ iss.

35. $6\frac{1}{4}$ L of 4% Lysol

36. 1.5%

37. 16.4 mL

38. 30 mL of 25% magnesium sulfate

39. ℳ x of the 0.05% solution

40. 3 L of 0.003% Merthiolate

41. Take 0.25 g of gentian violet and add enough rubbing alcohol to make exactly 25 mL.

42. Take 1.5 g of hydrocortisone and add enough lotion to make exactly 300 mL.

43. 31.5 oz sterile water

44. 2%; 1:50

45. Take 100 g of potassium permanganate crystals and add enough sterile solvent to make exactly 0.5 L.

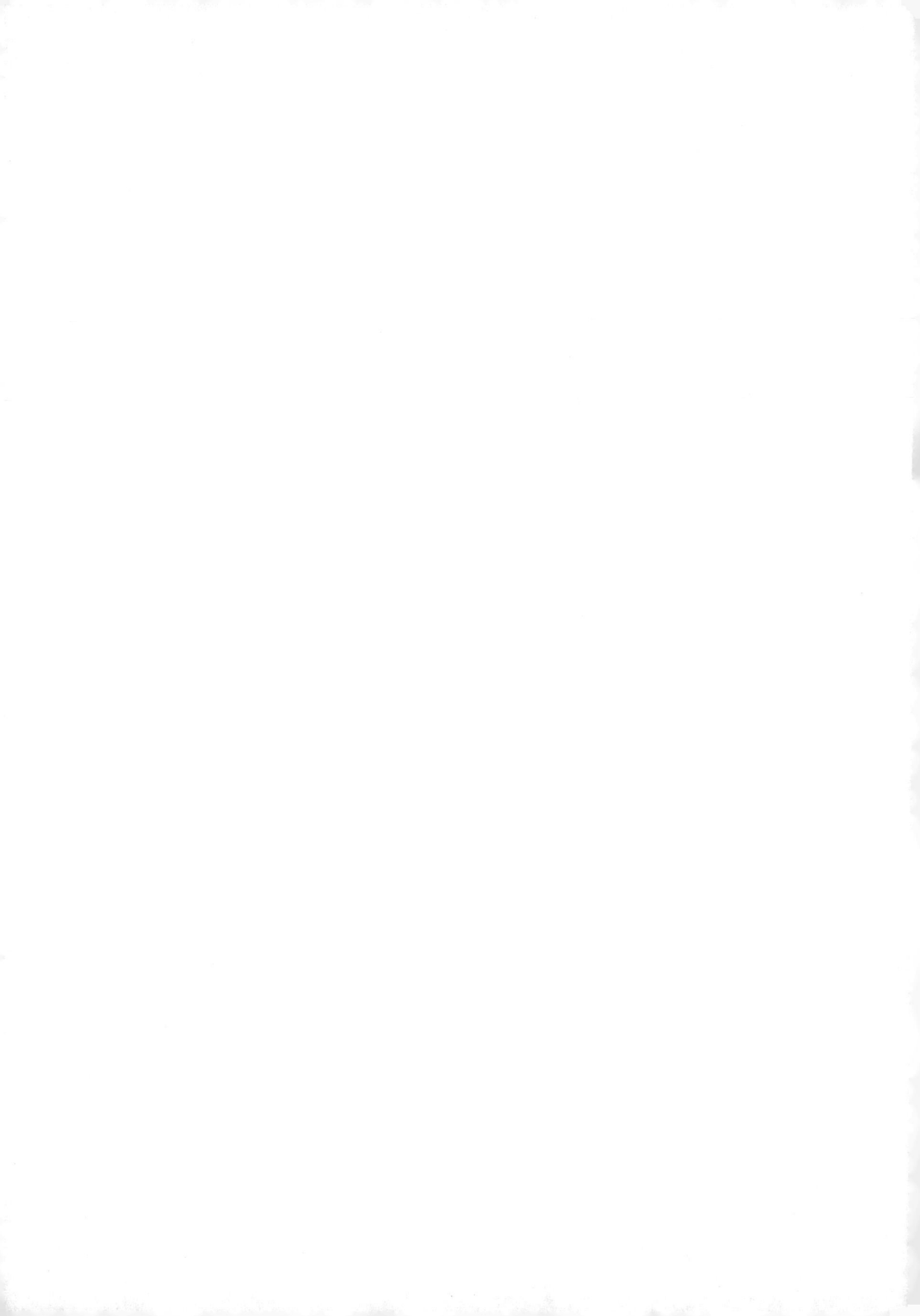